W9-BHG-422

Healthy Living

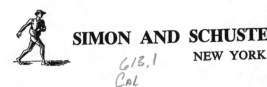

SIMON AND SCHUSTER
NEW YORK

in an Unhealthy World

Edward J. Calabrese
and Michael W. Dorsey

Copyright © 1984 by Edward Calabrese and Michael Dorsey
All rights reserved
including the right of reproduction
in whole or in part in any form
Published by Simon and Schuster
A Division of Simon & Schuster, Inc.
Simon & Schuster Building
Rockefeller Center
1230 Avenue of the Americas
New York, New York 10020

SIMON AND SCHUSTER and colophon are registered trademarks
of Simon & Schuster, Inc.
Designed by Irving Perkins Associates
Manufactured in the United States of America

1 2 3 4 5 6 7 8 9 10

Library of Congress Cataloging in Publication Data

Calabrese, Edward J., date.
    Healthy living in an unhealthy world.

    Bibliography: p.
    Includes index.
    1. Environmental health.   2. Nutrition.
3. Environmentally induced diseases—Nutritional
aspects.   4. Pollution—Toxicology.   I. Dorsey,
Michael W.   II. Title.
RA566.C26   1984   613′.1   83-14754
ISBN 0-671-44759-9

Contents |

Illustrations |

Tables

Figures

Preface |

A few years ago, one of the coauthors of this book, Edward J. Calabrese, Ph.D., wrote a two-volume work for the scientific and medical communities. In over 1,000 pages, *Nutrition and Environmental Health* (John Wiley and Sons, 1980 and 1981) provided the first comprehensive overview of a new branch of the sciences of nutrition and public health—a branch that explores the effects of diet on one's susceptibility to hazardous substances in the environment. From the reaction to that book and from subsequent talks with scientists and nonscientists alike, it became apparent that the subject of nutrient-pollutant interactions is of interest to a great many people.

It has become increasingly apparent over the past few decades that the environment is the leading cause of human sickness. In particular, major killers like cancer and heart disease have been tied to such environmental agents as radiation, manmade industrial pollutants, medications and diet. The more scientists have searched, the greater the number of hazardous substances they have found lurking in our food, our air, our drinking water, our homes and the tissues of our bodies. There is simply no way to escape these ubiquitous pollutants and lead a normal life.

It is little wonder, then, that some Americans have taken a fatalistic approach to life. "If one thing doesn't get you, something else will" is an often-heard reason for giving up and allowing oneself to become a victim of a potentially hazardous environment. But, instead of giving up, many people have looked for ways to gain control over the environment and over their lives. This book is about a science that is already beginning to place that control

11

in everyone's hands. But, as you will read in Chapter 1, it is not complete control, not the ultimate answer. We do not describe in this book a miracle cure or a quick fix.

Instead, this book will introduce you to a growing body of research that is just beginning to have an important effect, for the better, on your life. Working as a team, the authors, a scientist and a science writer, have translated a massive and rapidly growing body of scientific literature concerning the effect of diet on environmental disease for a nontechnical audience. The art of translation is a delicate one. Scientists speak a precise and highly technical language. Writing that is clear and meaningful to them is often full of jargon and too difficult to understand for everyone else. On the other hand, works of science for the general public are sometimes too simplistic, misleading or vague for the scientific sensibility. The science writer must walk a tightrope between these two audiences, risking oversimplification on the one hand and confusion on the other.

We believe our complementary skills as scientist and science writer have allowed us to successfully negotiate this high wire. We believe we have produced a book that has the objectivity required of careful science writing but that is not shy about explaining what this new field of science might mean to readers and how they can apply its findings in their own lives. We think it is a work that will interest and be enjoyed by scientists and all the rest of us.

We would like to thank Linda Carli and Mary Calabrese for reading portions of the manuscript and assuring us that our sometimes tentative steps were indeed taking us closer to the end of that tightrope. We would also like to thank Natalie Banack and Craig Forni for their help in preparing the figures and tables.

EDWARD J. CALABRESE
Amherst, Massachusetts

MICHAEL DORSEY
Belchertown, Massachusetts

CHAPTER 1

A Science in the Making:
Nutrition and Environmental Health

It has been said that what you don't know can't hurt you. Unfortunately, what you are not aware of can hurt you and, in fact, already has. The odds are one in four that you will get cancer in your lifetime. The chances are greater than one in six that you will die from cancer. If you escape cancer, there are more than enough other premature ills to go around—heart disease, kidney disorders, emphysema, anemia and liver disease, to name just a few.

The causes of these diseases, in nearly all cases, are in the environment. We live in a tainted world. The air we breathe, the water we drink, the food we eat and the buildings in which we live and work are contaminated with the by-products of our modern world. It is virtually impossible to avoid these omnipresent chemicals. Even the book you are now reading will leave minute traces on your hands of the inks, glues and other chemicals used to make it.

Unfortunately, we don't yet know how great a risk we encounter from the environment in our daily lives. Of the hundreds of chemicals that surround us, some are highly toxic. Some cause cancer and many others are suspected carcinogens. Taking them one at a time, scientists can often estimate the health risks they pose. But we are not exposed to one chemical at a time. We spend our entire lives in a complex brew of substances that interact in unknown ways to affect our lives and health. Sorting out these interactions and determining how risky our lives are is like putting together a jigsaw puzzle with a nearly infinite number of pieces.

The chemical sea around us is kept in check to a limited degree by a sea wall of legislation and regulations administered by a handful of federal and state agencies. For instance, the 1976 federal Toxic Substances Control Act, one of the more ambitious pieces of legislation aimed at protecting Americans from hazardous substances, requires manufacturers to provide the government with experimental data explaining the effects new chemicals will likely have on the public. In addition, the United States Environmental Protection Agency (EPA) has the power to ban chemicals now in circulation if they are deemed an unacceptable threat to public health. The Food and Drug Administration (FDA) and the Department of Agriculture (USDA) have similar powers for certain classes of compounds.

A major problem, however, is enforcement. With too few inspectors, too few technicians and insufficient funds, the agencies that must see that the laws and regulations are followed are often not entirely up to the task. In addition, assessing the safety of even a single chemical can be a costly and time-consuming process. Considering the number of new substances that are offered for review each year, it is not surprising that only a small number of compounds have been adequately tested.

Because of the staggering cost of thoroughly studying new chemicals and evaluating the safety of substances already liberally spread throughout our environment, and because of the incomprehensible difficulty of ridding the environment of agents that could potentially harm human beings, there is a growing acceptance among scientists and government regulators that exposure to these hazards cannot be eliminated. We must continue to live our lives among a bewildering number of poisonous and carcinogenic agents.

If we cannot avoid the hazards of our environment, can we at least increase our resistance to them and reduce our odds of succumbing to the diseases they cause? Are we doomed to remain helpless victims of a swelling sea of harmful substances, or is there a way we can reduce our susceptibility to the chemical insults in our surroundings?

A growing body of evidence suggests that we can indeed reduce the risks the environment presents. The tool that can give us that control is simple and within our grasp. It is nutrition. The foods we eat—the vitamins, minerals and other nutrients we consume—may have a profound effect on our chances of getting cancer and many other environmentally induced diseases. Nutrition, in short, holds the promise of becoming a significant weapon in the fight against pollution and other hazards in our world.

But the science of nutrition and environmental health is a new field. Many of its conclusions are tentative and in need of further testing. What we are presenting in this book is an early glimpse of a science in the making. Our goal is to introduce you to this new field, which is just beginning to explore the ways in which nutrients interact with environmental agents. How you use the information that follows is ultimately up to you.

Americans have already been bombarded with an overwhelming amount of advice about nutrition. Nutrition books cram the shelves in bookstores. Many newspapers now run regular columns on the subject. Radio and television talk-shows buzz with the topic, and several entire magazines are devoted to spreading the good word about food. Nutrition, we are told, can cure the common cold, lengthen our lives, increase our sexual vigor and make us healthier, stronger, more attractive and more interesting people. If ever there was a panacea, nutrition must be it.

Most of these claims have been incompletely or poorly tested, if they have been tested at all. Science is a strict discipline, and scientists are a largely skeptical crowd. Before something can be said to be true beyond a reasonable scientific doubt, it must stand up to close scrutiny and criticism. Nutrition gurus, health food proponents and megavitamin advocates rarely have such high standards.

So you will not find unreasonable claims in this book, just the facts. You will find no quick fixes and no miracle diets. You will, however, find information you can use right now to help you begin leading a healthier life. In many cases, the findings of this new area of nutritional science have been well tested and have survived the critical spotlight of scientific review. For example we know that:

—Vitamin C eaten along with a meal of cured meat or bacon can prevent the formation of potent carcinogens known as nitrosamines.

—Pectin, a fiber found in apples and other fruit, can markedly reduce the amount of lead the human body absorbs from the environment.

—Vitamin E prevents the damage air pollutants such as ozone can do to the lungs.

—Vitamin A in its natural forms and in new synthetic analogs may prevent and cure cancers caused by many environmental agents.

We will tell you what is known, what is suspected and what may become known with further research. We will probably pose more questions than we answer, but this is the nature of science.

The findings described in this book may have far-reaching implications. The more scientists learn about the effects of the food we eat on our susceptibility to environmental hazards, the more they are discovering the inadequacy of our current government policies regarding nutrition. To date, the methodology used to determine the standard daily requirement for various nutrients does not consider the value of many of these nutrients in fighting environmental pollution. Amounts of certain nutrients that will maintain health and prevent deficiency diseases may not be enough to shield us from agents in the environment. Consequently, our entire approach to determining Recommended Dietary Allowances (RDAs) may have to be rethought. When standards are set for safe levels of pollutants and industrial chemicals, it is rarely considered that common nutritional deficiencies can markedly enhance the susceptibility of the human body to these chemical agents. What may be safe for an adult who eats a balanced diet may be toxic or even carcinogenic to someone who has poor nutrition. Our government policies in this area also seem due for an overhaul.

The information in the heart of this book, Chapters 5 through 9, was distilled from hundreds of articles and books by scientists working in the field of environmental health. The topics covered were gleaned from research by nutritionists, public health scientists, toxicologists, epidemiologists, physiologists, microbiologists and many other scientists. Each of these five chapters deals with a different class of hazardous agents. Chapters 5 and 6 deal with chemicals that are difficult, if not impossible, to avoid—those in our food, air, water and land. Chapters 7 and 8 discuss chemicals in medications and those we encounter on the job. These are substances that we can avoid, but only at the possible risk of poor health or by changing professions. Chapter 9 covers agents we deliberately expose ourselves to, such as alcohol and the numerous toxic and carcinogenic chemicals in cigarette smoke. Also in Chapter 9 we deal with fads and lifestyles that can affect our susceptibility to pollutants and other environmental agents.

For many of you, the subjects covered in these chapters will be unfamiliar. To help you understand the research you will read about in Chapters 5 through 9, we have provided brief introductions to nutrition and to the sciences of toxicology and epidemiology in Chapters 3 and 4. We think these provide interesting and useful synopses. Many readers may also not be familiar with the units of measure commonly used by scientists. While most Americans continue to use the English system of measurement, scientists the world over have adopted the more precise and more logical metric system. This book reflects the split between scientists and laymen; you will find both systems represented. Where possible, we have expressed things in ounces, inches and so on. However, this was not always possible. For those who feel uncomfortable with meters and liters and grams, here is a quick guide to the metric system:

PREFIXES: The metric system uses a standard set of prefixes to denote fractions and multiples of several standard units:

> Kilo —one thousand
> Hecto—one hundred
> Deca —ten
> Deci —one tenth
> Centi —one hundredth
> Milli —one thousandth
> Micro—one millionth

The prefixes you will see most often in this book are *kilo, milli* and *micro.*

VOLUME: The standard metric unit of volume is the liter. A liter is slightly larger than a quart. Water pollution standards are usually expressed in so much of a substance per liter of water. Smaller volumes are usually expressed in terms of milliliters. This is equal to one thousandth of a liter, or about four hundredths of a fluid ounce (just about 20 drops from an eyedropper).

WEIGHT: The metric unit of weight is the gram. There are about 28 grams in an ounce. The packets of sugar provided in restaurants each weigh just over 2.5 grams. As small as a gram is, it is not small enough to measure the quantities of pollutants found in the environment or the amount of nutrients we must consume each day. So scientists typically speak in terms of milligrams, which are thousandths of a gram, and micrograms, which are millionths of a gram.

To measure larger weights, such as the body weights of animals or people, scientists use the kilogram, which is 1,000 grams, or 2.2 pounds. A 150-pound man weighs about 68 kilograms.

LENGTH: The meter is the metric unit of length. One meter equals just over a yard. For small lengths, scientists use the millimeter, which is one thousandth of a meter.

PARTS OF SPEECH: Sometimes pollution standards are expressed in parts per million or parts per billion. These terms are like the commonly used expression percent, which actually means parts per hundred.

We hope you find the information in the chapters that follow interesting and useful. But, most of all, we hope it opens your eyes, not only to the potential of nutrition to prevent and cure environmental disease, but to the immensity of the problem of hazardous substances and agents in the environment. To give you an idea of the magnitude of that problem, in the next chapter we'll look at the staggering number of toxic and carcinogenic agents one may encounter in a single day.

CHAPTER 2

Surviving in a Polluted World:
A Short Story

In two homes 80 miles apart, alarm clocks sound the start of a hot, muggy summer day. One clock buzzes in the bedroom of a town house in Boston's Back Bay area. Rachel Burgess stretches and switches off the clock as she and her husband, Tom, rise to face another day.

In Storrs, Connecticut, an academic community surrounded by green, rolling hills and farms, another clock announces the morning with the 6:00 A.M. news. While sunlight streams in through the window and the thermometer begins to rise, John and Laura Hill pull themselves out of bed.

In the next 16 hours, these four people will spend a fairly typical day. They will work at their jobs, eat three meals, attend to household chores, indulge in pastimes and spend about an hour each riding in cars or public transportation. Also, like most of us, they will encounter a few thousand poisonous, mutagenic and carcinogenic chemicals before they settle down to bed this evening. These couples are fictional, but the arsenal of potentially hazardous substances they will encounter today is real. These are, indeed, the same chemicals most of us are likely to meet in an average day.

Even as these couples slept, they were breathing in a potentially toxic substance: dust. Along with its usual components—soil, bacteria and mold—dust contains the remnants of our lifestyles. Propellants from aerosol cans, fumes from household solvents and cleaners, carcinogens from cigarette smoke, radioactive radon gas from concrete and other earthen building materials, and many other substances can attach themselves to particles of dust. In a modern, well-insulated home like the Hills', airborne substances may build up to levels that exceed the federal limits for acceptable occupational exposure, especially during cold weather when homes are sealed up.

In the Burgesses' apartment the dust carries with it an unhealthy dose of common city air pollutants. Lead from cars burning leaded gasoline, asbestos from brake linings, sulfur dioxide from nearby oil-fired power plants and gaseous hydrocarbons from vehicle exhaust and industries mingle with the other dust particles in the air.

During the winter, dust is even more of a hazard. When it falls on hot surfaces, such as the cooking range, the furnace in the Burgesses' basement or the woodstove the Hills installed last year, some of the organic compounds it carries can react to form minute but detectable quantities of phosgene and hydrogen cyanide, two toxic gases.

The two couples rise and begin their morning routines. Rachel Burgess steps into the shower and turns on the water. While she bathes, vinyl chloride, a known human carcinogen, enters the air from a new shower curtain, the lighting fixtures and the bathmat. A small organic molecule, vinyl chloride is linked into chains to form the common plastic polyvinyl chloride (PVC), which is used for weatherstripping, footwear, upholstery, records, car seats, garden hose, credit cards, food wrappers and water pipe. In concentrations much higher than the dose Rachel receives in her bathroom this morning, vinyl chloride can damage the liver, skin, bones and lungs. The most serious problem with vinyl chloride, though, is its ability to produce a rare form of liver cancer (see Chapter 7). The effects of low-level, daily exposure over many years beginning soon after birth, the kind of exposure most people receive, are not fully understood.

After her shower, Rachel sprays on an antiperspirant. Nearly all such products contain aluminum salts. Rachel's brand is made with aluminum chlorhydrate. Aluminum salts replaced zirconium salts in the mid-1970s after the latter were taken off the market by the FDA because they may cause granulomas (hard lumps in the armpits) in a small number of individuals and because they caused lung tumors in laboratory animals when sprayed into the air with aerosol propellants. So far, the only proven health effect of aluminum salts is a skin irritation that can occur in hypersensitive individuals, although they are being evaluated to see if they, too, damage the lungs.

Rachel also sprinkles on some talcum powder before getting dressed. Talc and asbestos are generally found in adjacent geological veins, and great care must be taken in mining and processing talc to prevent talcum products from becoming contaminated with asbestos, which has been linked to a form of human lung cancer. Although most talc powders marketed in the United States are relatively free of asbestos, it is nearly impossible to produce completely uncontaminated talc. In a study conducted at Brigham and Women's Hospital in Boston, it was found that women who used talc on their genitals and sanitary napkins were three times as likely to develop ovarian cancer as women who did not use talc. It is not known how talc is related to the onset of cancer or whether the talc these women used contained asbestos. But by itself, talc is not known to be a carcinogen.

At the Hill home, Laura slips into a new cotton jumpsuit while her husband buttons up a new permanent-press shirt. Most no-iron clothing is treated with formaldehyde. Manufacturers soak permanent-press fabrics in an aqueous solution made with this colorless, pungent gas to give the cloth body. Unfortunately, residues of the formaldehyde remain in the cloth after manufacture and escape into the air to be inhaled by the wearer. In fact, some of the t-shirts Laura recently bought had a disagreeable odor when she first purchased them. Formaldehyde, which is also found in shampoo, mascara, toothpaste, draperies, tissues, air fresheners and many other products, can cause nasal cancer in mice and rats and is a suspected human carcinogen. While Laura and John are probably not exposed to enough of this chemical in their home to be at significant risk of cancer, the story is quite different for the residents of a mobile home park near their house.

Mobile homes often consist of a small, poorly ventilated space largely surrounded by walls, floors, ceilings, furniture, carpeting and even insulation constructed of plywood, particle board and other products made with formaldehyde. Toxic levels of formaldehyde gas, levels high enough to induce cancer in laboratory animals, have been detected in some of these homes. High levels have also been found in houses insulated with urea formaldehyde foam insulation, which was banned in 1982 by the Consumer Product Safety Commission.

After dressing, Laura puts on her makeup. Her lipstick contains a coal-tar dye. Several of these dyes, which are also found in hair coloring, are known carcinogens in laboratory animals and some, such as Red Dye No. 2, have been banned. Laura also applies nail polish that contains butyl acetate, a toxic chemical that has been known to irritate the eyes, split nails and occasionally turn the skin under the nails black if used too frequently. Formaldehyde, the main ingredient in the nail hardener Laura keeps in her cosmetic case, can damage cuticles and numb the fingertips if overused.

Before leaving the bathroom, Laura applies a quick shot of hair spray. Like many aerosol products, hair sprays contain fluorocarbon propellants, which in large doses can cause nausea, loss of consciousness, liver damage and even lung cancer. Fluorocarbons are particularly dangerous in hair sprays, which are normally used near the nose and mouth. Because of their small size, the propellants are readily absorbed into the bloodstream if inhaled, possibly carrying other components of the spray into the blood along with them. In addition to propellants, hair sprays contain plasticizers, solvents, alcohol, shellac, silicones and scents, many of which are inherently toxic to biological tissues.

In both homes, the time has come for breakfast. Rachel, a light eater, sips a cup of tea sweetened with saccharin and munches on a piece of toast spread with peanut butter. Tom, who rarely eats breakfast, just has coffee today. The Hills have always believed in big breakfasts. This morning Laura cooks bacon and eggs, which she and John wash down with orange juice.

Rachel's tea and Tom's coffee, along with many other foods and over-the-counter medicines, contain caffeine. A central nervous system stimulant and a diuretic, caffeine is known to cause a number of minor health problems, including rapid heartbeat, heartburn and anxiety. In various studies, caffeine has been found to induce mutations, heart disease and bladder cancer, but these findings have not been confirmed. Dr. Brian MacMahon and his associates at the Harvard School of Public Health linked coffee-drinking to cancer of the pancreas, but the causative agent does not appear to be caffeine, since similar results were not obtained with tea.

Rachel is two months pregnant. There is considerable disagreement about whether caffeine will pose a risk to the child she is carrying. Various studies have found that caffeine can reduce fertility and promote birth defects. The risk of miscarriage, premature births and stillbirths has also been shown to be higher in women who are heavy coffee drinkers, although a recent study by scientists at Harvard University of 12,205 women at Brigham and Women's Hospital in Boston found no relationship between coffee-drinking and low birth weights, premature deliveries or birth defects. However, women who, like Rachel, reported smoking three or more cigarettes a day seemed more likely to give birth to underweight babies. It is possible that smoking may have biased results of previous studies. Another study of the mothers of over 2,000 malformed infants at the Boston University Drug Epidemiology Unit also found no relationship between caffeine and birth defects. However, in a study of a large group of white, middle-class women, Dr. Sandra Jacobson, a psychologist at Wayne State University, found that nonsmoking women who consume six to seven cups of coffee a day had infants who exhibited poor neuromuscular and reflex functions and signs of physical immaturity (which, according to Jacobson, they may outgrow).

The official verdict is also out on saccharin, the artificial sweetener commonly added to diet foods and soft drinks. Rachel puts saccharin in hot drinks and also uses it instead of sugar in puddings and in other desserts that do not require cooking or baking. Several studies conducted since the 1950s have found a link between the sweetener and bladder cancer in laboratory animals. In 1977, a study by Canadian scientists showed that bladder cancer occurred in male offspring of pregnant rats fed large doses of saccharin, leading to a ban on saccharin in Canada and an unsuccessful attempt by the United States FDA to halt its use in this country. Epidemiological studies have not yet provided conclusive proof that saccharin can cause cancer in people.

Peanut butter, an American staple, contains an extremely potent carcinogen known as aflatoxin. Produced by *Aspergillus flavus,* a mold that grows on peanuts, corn and certain grains, as little as a billionth of a gram of aflatoxin eaten each day can increase one's chance of getting liver cancer. Although peanuts used for peanut butter in this country are carefully checked for *Aspergillus* growth, it is virtually impossible to produce aflatoxin-free peanut products and, in fact, the FDA now permits up to 20 parts per billion aflatoxin in peanut butter.

The bacon on the Hills' plates, along with other cured meats (pepperoni, sausages, cold cuts and so on) and smoked fish, contains a food additive known as sodium nitrite. Sodium nitrite has a characteristic taste and prevents the growth of bacteria that produce the deadly botulism toxin. Nitrites can combine with a type of organic chemicals in food known as amines to form nitrosamines, some of the most potent cancer-causing substances known. The reaction between nitrites and amines can occur when the food is cooked or processed or when the two ingredients mix in the acidic environment of the stomach right after a meal.

Meats and fish are not the only sources of nitrites. The majority of the nitrites we consume are formed naturally in our saliva. In addition, nitrates in vegetables and in drinking water contaminated with runoff from fertilized fields may be converted to nitrites in the stomachs of infants. Nitrosamines themselves are found in many beers and scotches.

The Burgesses leave their apartment and board a crosstown bus for the start of their daily trek to work. During the 20-minute ride they will breathe in the air of the city, which on the best of days is an unhealthy conglomeration of pollutants. The bulk of this complex mixture is contributed by motor vehicles, industry, power plants, oil-fired furnaces and incinerators.

As they travel into the center of the city, Rachel and Tom are breathing in a noxious blend of carbon monoxide, which binds strongly with the hemoglobin in their red blood cells; sulfur dioxide and nitrogen dioxide, which irritate their eyes and throats; and ozone, which makes their throats feel scratchy. Ozone is commonly found during the summer wherever auto traffic is high, as it is today in Boston. In Los Angeles where cars are the principal means of transportation, ozone levels have been known to rise to four times the EPA ambient air quality standard. Ozone, also produced by photocopy machines and welding operations can aggravate respiratory problems and has been shown to age the skin and lungs and increase the risk of lung cancer and chromosomal abnormalities. It is a special danger to the elderly and to athletes who exercise in city air.

While they ride the bus to work, Rachel and Tom breathe in fumes from the bus and other vehicles. The fumes contain a host of toxic and carcinogenic compounds, some of which come from the additives blended with gasoline and diesel fuel to prevent knocking, combat engine deposits and reduce the corrosion of engine parts. The antiknock agent tetraethyl lead is still an important source of lead in the environment. Diesel exhaust, like that from the bus the Burgesses are traveling in, contains more particulates and more oxides of nitrogen than the exhaust from gasoline engines. Diesel exhaust is also more likely to cause mutations than gasoline exhaust.

Compounds spewing out of tailpipes are not hazards only as air pollutants. Emissions from cars and trucks, which also include barium, zinc, phosphorus and the nervous system toxin tricresyl phosphate, are deposited on the surfaces of roads. Flushed by rain, these compounds become important water pollutants and sometimes contaminate reservoirs that lie near roads and highways.

The constituents of exhaust can combine with one another and with other components of air pollution, especially when exposed to sunlight, to form other, potentially more hazardous substances. For example, a study by Hiroshi Tokiwa and his colleagues at the Fukuoka Environmental Research Center in Japan found that particulate matter in air pollution can combine with nitrogen dioxide, nitric acid and sulfur dioxide in auto exhaust to form mutagenic compounds.

Although less polluted, the air in the Hills' Connecticut town is far from pristine. We know this because a team of researchers from the National Institute for Occupational Safety and Health accidentally discovered that country air is not always as clean as it seems. Preparing for a study of airborne mutagens in the workplace, they mounted an air sampler on the roof of their Morgantown, West Virginia, lab to collect baseline data. Expecting to find little or no mutagenic activity, the researchers were surprised to learn that the air in Morgantown, a relatively rural community, was five to seven times as mutagenic as filtered air. The researchers believed the mutagens had drifted in from Pittsburgh and other industrial centers 60 or more miles away, leading them to wonder whether any area of the country can escape air pollution.

As if city air were not enough, Rachel Burgess creates her own air pollution by smoking cigarettes. The smoke from her cigarettes contains numerous poisons and cancer-causing substances. Formaldehyde, benzo(a)pyrene, nitrosamines, nicotine, carbon monoxide, cyanide, lead, cadmium, ammonia and a variety of radioactive compounds constitute only a partial list of the substances in each puff of the cigarette Rachel is now smoking. Each time she inhales the smoke, she breathes these pollutants deep into the passages of her lungs. Here they pass into the bloodstream or, mixed with sticky tars, remain trapped in the air sacs, greatly increasing Rachel's risk of developing lung cancer, emphysema and cardiovascular disease.

Smoke is not only a threat to people who voluntarily light up cigarettes and breathe in the poisonous effluent. Nonsmokers who by misfortune happen to be in the same room, car, crowded elevator or city bus with a smoker also inhale the toxic waste and may suffer the same health effects. Especially at risk are spouses and children of smokers. Resha Putzrath and other scientists at the Harvard School of Public Health studied the mutagenic activity of urine from smokers and nonsmokers. Compounds in cigarette smoke are carried by the blood to the kidneys, and subsequently to the bladder. This may be one reason smokers have an increased incidence of bladder cancer. Putzrath found mutagens in the urine from all of the smokers, but only one nonsmoker had mutagenic urine. That person was the only nonsmoker married to a smoker.

Like many pregnant women, Rachel will continue to smoke and drink while she carries her child. Studies have suggested that mothers who smoke have a one-third greater chance of delivering their infants stillborn. Women who drink fare little better. A pregnant woman who drinks 2 ounces of alcohol a day (about three mixed drinks, three 6-ounce glasses of wine or three 12-ounce bottles of beer) runs an increased risk of having a child with a group of birth defects known as fetal alcohol syndrome, which includes a deformed face, poor muscle development and improperly formed heart and brain. Drinking only twice a week increases the risk of miscarriage, according to a study by the National Institute of Child Health and Human Development. Smoking and drinking have also both been linked to undersized infants.

Alcohol, of course, has a variety of other negative health effects, even for light drinkers. It dilates blood vessels, injures kidney cells and can destroy cells of the liver and brain. Alcohol use also seems to increase one's risk of cancer, especially for heavy drinkers and particularly for those who both smoke and drink heavily. Imbibing two to three drinks a day can double one's risk of oral cancer, but drinking that amount and smoking two packs a day increases one's oral cancer risk 15 times.

Tom Burgess is an artist and art instructor. He and several other artists own a small studio in the heart of Boston and together they practice and teach a variety of art techniques. Though art is not usually considered a hazardous occupation, a look at the cabinets and storeroom in an average studio might change one's opinion. Artists use a surprising variety of chemicals, some found typically in industry. They are often used carelessly, by industrial standards, in poorly ventilated, cramped rooms.

Paints are made up of media that can contain ammonia, formaldehyde and benzene; pigments that can contain such heavy-metal toxins as lead, mercury and cadmium and such known and suspected carcinogens as barium chromate, lamp black, chromic oxide, copper arsenite, strontium chromate and zinc chromate; and preservatives, which can contain mercury. Printmakers use toxic lead and magnesium driers; concentrated tannic, nitric and phosphoric acids for etching stones; and liquid asphalt, which may cause skin cancer. Those who work with ceramics can breathe in powdered aluminum silicate clay, which can cause a debilitating lung disease known as silicosis. Sculptors can be exposed to silica and asbestos dust, which can cause lung tumors, and welders can encounter carbon monoxide and skin-cancer-inducing ultraviolet light. The photographic darkroom is a storehouse of toxins too numerous to mention.

As a sales representative for a major chemical company, Rachel frequently visits industrial plants, businesses and other facilities to take orders and answer inquiries from customers. Her first stop today is a stainless-steel manufacturing plant where workers are exposed to chromium dust, which can cause respiratory problems, pain on breathing, headaches and loss of weight, and iron dust, which can cause lung irritations and cancer when mixed with silica, radioactive materials or ferric oxide. At many of the installations Rachel visits, she and workers are exposed to an amazing variety of toxic and cancer-causing chemicals. For example, at a second factory she will visit today, workers handle styrene, a plastics building block that can irritate the lungs and possibly cause cancer, and benzene, which has been linked to leukemia in chronically exposed workers.

In the afternoon, Rachel visits a small private hospital. While there, she chats with two operating-room nurses who tell her they occasionally feel dizzy and experience headaches and nausea after their shifts. Rachel suggests having the ventilation systems in the operating rooms checked. If these malfunction, anesthetic fumes and other chemicals can build up. In epidemiological studies, operating-room personnel have been found to incur a higher than average incidence of cancer and spontaneous abortions and were more likely to give birth to children with congenital defects. Many researchers have attributed this to exposure to inhalation anesthetics such as halothane, a compound that is known to be mutagenic.

Reproductive abnormalities, such as birth defects, stillbirths and spontaneous abortions, are occupational hazards in many professions. The developing fetus may be extremely sensitive to chemical insults, such as the mutagens and carcinogens found in numerous businesses and industries. Dealing with this threat to the unborn is an immense and challenging problem. Efforts to reduce worker exposure to chemicals have helped, but have not eliminated the problem. Barring women of childbearing age from the workplace would, of course, be ludicrous. The solution is not to eliminate workers who are at high risk, but to lower or eliminate the risk.

In Connecticut, the Hills are also spending an average day at work. Laura is a secretary at a nearby college; John is a maintenance worker at the same school. As a secretary, Laura inhales, contacts and ingests a variety of toxins. For example, during the morning, she breathes in ozone, an air pollutant, while photocopying a large report. Copying machines give off appreciable amounts of ozone, which, in poorly ventilated rooms, can sometimes exceed the OSHA standard of industrial exposure of no more than 0.1 part per million for an eight-hour average.

Secretaries and other clerical workers are also exposed to solvents, inks, paper, duplicating fluids, type cleaners, correction fluids, ink removers and carbon paper, all of which contain toxic or carcinogenic agents.

As a maintenance worker, John must handle pesticides and herbicides, two of the most insidious types of environmental pollutants. Because of their widespread use by farmers, power companies and home gardeners, they often pollute our waterways, our land, our food and our bodies. As the population continues to grow, so do the use, abuse, number and complexity of these compounds.

Among the pest killers John must handle are several highly toxic herbicides, such as 2,4-D and paraquat, which have been linked to cancer in animals; strychnine, a highly toxic rodent killer; hydrogen cyanide, an extremely poisonous fumigant; and insecticides. Not long ago, most insecticides were chlorinated compounds that killed insects effectively but were not highly toxic to people. But these compounds, including the widely used DDT, were found to be very persistent in the environment, hanging around for generations and passing up the food chain to become concentrated in higher animals, including people. Chlorinated compounds have been largely replaced by organic phosphate pesticides. These are more biodegradable, but are also much more toxic to people. Such compounds as malathion, parathion, diazinon and Ethion cause symptoms ranging from dizziness and headaches to convulsions, depending on the amount ingested.

Pest killers are not the only chemicals John deals with in his job. Today he tunes a pool car engine, inhaling carbon monoxide and the other substances in auto exhaust. He also changes the oil. Waste oil contains a variety of heavy metals such as lead, barium, zinc and phosphorus. Oil fresh from the can is laced with toxic organic additives designed to improve the performance of engines.

For his lunch, John stops at a nearby coffee shop for a hamburger. Ground beef, another American staple, is also a good source of substances one would expect to find only in a pharmacy. Cattle raisers feed a number of antibiotics, tranquilizers, enzymes and hormones to their animals to make them fatten up quicker, stay calm, lose their sex drive and produce tender meat. The widespread consumption of antibiotics in meat is now thought to be helping to promote the evolution of antibiotic-resistant strains of disease-causing bacteria. The full effects on health of another common beef additive, diethylstilbestrol, or DES, are uncertain, although DES is known to have caused cervical and testicular cancer in a small percentage of the daughters and sons of mothers who took DES in the past to prevent miscarriages.

When a hamburger is fried on a grill or in a frying pan, mutagens are produced. Several studies have found that when ground beef is fried at 200° F until well done, substances, as yet unidentified, will form that will cause mutations in bacterial assays. John Weisburger, of the American Health Foundation, has postulated that some of these mutagens may act selectively on the lower digestive tract. A cooperative research project mounted by Japanese and United States scientists is seeking to identify the mutagens, using over a ton of fried hamburger.

Laura pauses at her desk for a tunafish sandwich. Tuna and several other varieties of marine and fresh-water fish contain mercury. The amount of mercury commonly found in the flesh of fish varies from species to species, but most marine fish are contaminated with between 0.1 and 0.15 part per million. Swordfish occasionally contains more than one part per million. Levels as high as 0.2 part per million are considered normal for many species of fresh-water fish.

Mercury is used in a variety of industrial applications, from the synthesis of chlorine to the manufacture of electrical switches and test equipment. It was also once an ingredient in pesticides and antifungal treatments for seeds, uses that may account for a large portion of the mercury present in the environment. The exact amount of mercury required to produce symptoms of poisoning seems to vary widely, making it difficult to determine what levels are unsafe. In any case, the quantities normally present in fish seem far too small to produce acute poisoning, but whether eating fish with high mercury levels frequently can contribute to chronic mercury poisoning is not yet known. Interestingly, though, people who follow certain diet programs that emphasize fish as a source of protein usually have higher levels of mercury in their blood than others.

Laura's sandwich also contains traces of lead. The can of tuna Laura opened this morning was sealed with lead solder. Also found in car exhaust, paint, pottery glazes and cigarette smoke, lead is an insidious poison. Large doses, greater than what we normally get from our drinking water, our air or our food, can accumulate in the body, causing such symptoms as irritability, stomach pains, anemia and, possibly, brain damage. Children are most susceptible to the effects of lead and are also most likely to accidentally ingest large amounts in contaminated dirt and paint chips. Recognizing the problem of lead in canned foods, the Food and Drug Administration in 1973 launched an effort to get the canning industry to reduce and, in time, eliminate their use of lead solder. That effort concentrated initially on canned condensed milk, which is used to make infant formulas, and the results were impressive. A similar, though more modest, drop in lead in other canned foods has also been achieved.

With her tuna sandwich, Laura has a small bag of potato chips. Potatoes contain natural toxins known as glycoalkaloids, which inhibit the activity of cholinesterase, an enzyme essential for the transmission of signals in the nervous system. There are many other naturally occurring toxins and carcinogens. Aflatoxin, found in peanut butter, was mentioned earlier. Estragole, found in tarragon and anise, has been found to induce liver tumors in laboratory rats and mice. Tannins in tea (they are also found widely in vegetables) have been linked to cancer of the esophagus and stomach. Citral, found in oranges and lemons, can keep the body from making use of vitamin A. These are just a few of the dozens of poisons naturally found in foods.

To top off his lunch, Tom Burgess munches on a candy bar that contains caramel. A study by H. F. Stich and his colleagues at the British Columbia Research Center found that many caramelized sugars are capable of causing mutations. Stich prepared caramels of sucrose, glucose, fructose, maltose and other sugars and found that all produced mutations in cultures of Chinese hamster ovary cells. The sugars induced mutations known as chromosome breaks and exchanges, although uncaramelized sugars had no such effect. Stich also tested commercial caramel powders, which are used to color colas, beer, gravy mixes, meat products and syrups, with similar results. The researchers say more work will be needed before it can be concluded that caramels pose a risk to humans.

Before returning home, Rachel keeps an appointment with her hairdresser. For the last five years, she has had her hair colored because it is beginning to gray. The hairdresser applies a coloring agent that contains coal-tar dyes, many of which are known carcinogens. Because of a quirk in the law, the FDA cannot ban these hair-coloring dyes, but can only require that they carry warning labels. Certain lead acetate dyes, used to color hair slowly, also cause cancer in laboratory animals.

On her way home, Laura stops to run a load of clothes through a coin-operated dry-cleaning machine. Tetrachloroethylene, a compound commonly used in these machines, can depress the central nervous system and is known to cause liver damage in industrial workers who are chronically exposed to it. Another common dry-cleaning chemical, trichloroethylene, has been linked to liver, kidney and heart damage. Both compounds are known animal carcinogens. Users of coin-op dry-cleaning machines are often exposed to vapors when the doors are opened to retrieve the clothes. Today, in fact, Laura notices that the clothes are still wet with the cleaning compounds when she unloads the machine.

Home once again, both couples sit down to dinner. John and Laura have steak (more fried beef), asparagus (more nitrates) and coffee (more caffeine). The Burgess dinner includes pepperoni pizza (nitrosamines) and cola (caramel, artificial flavors and colors and caffeine). After dinner there is time for housework and other diversions. Laura polishes the dining-room furniture with a product that contains oil of cedarwood, a nervous system stimulant, and petroleum distillates and petroleum naphtha, two skin and respiratory tract irritants. She then washes a load of laundry with a detergent that contains a complex collection of toxins, skin irritants and caustic agents.

While Laura does the laundry, John cleans the oven with a product that contains lye, a caustic agent that can burn skin, eyes and the digestive tract. The cleaner also contains ammonia, another skin and eye irritant. Tripolyphosphate, another powerful skin irritant, is in the coffeepot cleaner John pours into the percolator.

At the Burgesses', the drain is clogged. Rachel uses a drain cleaner made from sulfuric acid. Tom Burgess is doing some remodeling work on the apartment. Tonight he is exposed to varying levels of lead, mercury and cadmium from old paint as he begins to tear down a wall. Later, he will encounter asbestos in spackling and patching compounds, possibly carcinogenic epoxy resins in glues, sawdust (a possible cause of nasal cancer) and phenol, an ingredient in paint remover that can irritate the eyes and damage the kidneys if ingested.

While Tom works, Rachel refinishes the bedroom furniture. The varnish remover she uses contains methylene chloride, a pleasant-smelling liquid that can dry the skin and irritate the eyes and upper respiratory tract. When inhaled, methylene chloride can enter the blood and react with red blood cells, forming a compound known as carboxyhemoglobin, which reduces the ability of blood to carry oxygen to the body's cells. Carbon monoxide in cigarette smoke can exacerbate the effects of methylene chloride. When Rachel, a smoker, and her husband, a nonsmoker, work on the refinishing together, Rachel feels dizzy within a few minutes, while Tom exhibits no noticeable effects.

Before they go to bed, the Burgesses turn on the bedroom air conditioner once more. While they sleep, minute amounts of the fluorocarbon refrigerant used in the machine drift through the bedroom. As they sleep, the Hills breath in radon, a radioactive gas found in concrete, bricks and other earthen materials. Radon tends to build up in well-insulated, poorly ventilated homes like the Hills' modern passive solar house.

In eight hours, both couples will awaken to spend another typical day in a world chock full of toxins, mutagens and carcinogens. In subsequent chapters, we will explain how nutrition can affect the way in which the body reacts to these hazardous chemicals. This information will constitute a synthesis of recent developments in the sciences of nutrition, toxicology and epidemiology, among others. Because these sciences are new to many people, Chapters 3 and 4 are designed to serve as primers on these exciting fields of research. They will help you understand the material that will follow.

CHAPTER 3

The Chemistry of Life: Nutrition

Like all matter, the human body is a complex collection of atoms and molecules. Chemicals allow us to move, think, speak and create new generations. Reciting a poem, kicking a football, laughing at a funny movie, recoiling from a frightening noise and digesting a gourmet meal all require the cooperation of many interlocking chemical systems.

Each chemical found in the human body plays one or more roles in the maintenance of life. The chemicals are organized into a complex architecture, at the center of which is the cell, the fundamental building block of all living things. The cell is like a living water balloon, but instead of a rubber skin, the cell is surrounded by a membrane—a chemical sandwich consisting of two layers of fats inside two layers of protein. Less than a hundred millionth of an inch thick, the cell membrane protects the cell and allows it to communicate with cells around it. It also acts as a selective barrier, letting food and oxygen in and waste out, but barring the passage of many other substances.

Inside the cell is a collection of tiny structures called organelles, which perform the cell's vital functions. At the center of the cells of higher animals and plants is an organelle known as the nucleus. Here, in long strands of a molecule called deoxyribonucleic acid, or DNA, is stored the cell's genetic blueprint. Every cell in the human body contains exactly the same information in its DNA as every other cell and has the potential to perform any of the body's functions, but each cell has its specialty. A cell's job is assigned to it while the body develops in the womb. By methods not yet understood, messages are sent to each new cell that shut down part of its genetic program and activate others. Thus, from the same general-purpose cell may be formed a muscle fiber or a nerve cell.

Groups of cells that perform the same functions are called tissues. Tissues of different types are organized into organs. The heart, for example, is made up of muscle tissue, blood vessels, nerve fibers and connective tissue (cells that hold the tissues of an organ together). Unlike tissues, which generally carry out only a few tasks, organs can often perform many functions. The liver is made up of cells that make blood-clotting chemicals, break down or destroy harmful substances and store food.

Organs are linked into systems, as the heart and blood vessels are organized into the cardiovascular system. The highest level of organization, systems perform the basic functions of life. The digestive system provides nourishment; the skeletal-muscular system allows the body to stand erect and move; the skin and immune systems protect the body from the outside world; and the urinary system removes wastes from the blood.

To perform these functions, the body's 40 trillion cells need a constant supply of energy and raw materials. Both come from food. When we eat, we supply our bodies with the chemicals they need to rebuild themselves, power their biological machinery and manufacture hundreds of essential substances. Among these are enzymes, substances that speed the progress of life-sustaining chemical reactions; hormones, the body's chemical messengers; and antibodies, chemicals that fight off infection and foreign matter.

To make use of the energy and raw materials in food, the body must first break the food down into its component parts. The digestive system, or gastrointestinal tract, is the body's food-processing plant. In this 15-foot-long tube, bite-sized portions of food are reduced in size and large molecules are broken down to forms that the body can use. Then the usable constituents are absorbed through the intestinal wall, literally moving from the outside of the body to the inside.

The process of digestion begins in the mouth, where the teeth chop and grind the food and mix it with saliva. Saliva moistens the food to ease its passage down the throat, and it contains an enzyme that begins converting starch into sugars. The food is then transported by waves of muscular contractions to the stomach.

The stomach breaks the food down a bit before it enters the remainder of the digestive tract. It also controls how fast the food moves into the small intestine, its next stop. Hydrochloric acid secreted by the stomach breaks down cell walls and loosens up the connective tissue that holds animal organs and tissues together, reducing the food to a thick soup called chyme. Pepsin, an enzyme secreted by glands in the stomach lining, chops proteins into smaller fragments. Other than small molecules like alcohol and aspirin, few substances are absorbed into the bloodstream from the stomach. After a few hours, the stomach muscles send the food into the small intestine.

In this nine-foot-long organ, proteins and carbohydrates receive their final processing. Here, enzymes supplied by the pancreas and bile salts from the liver go to work on the food and reduce it to a form that can be readily absorbed. The walls of the small intestine are lined with cells called villi, which project into the intestine, greatly increasing its surface area. In fact, if stretched out, the intestine could cover about 2,000 square feet, about the area of a singles tennis court.

All this surface area is necessary to absorb adequate amounts of nutrients as the food passes through the intestine. The villi are liberally supplied with blood vessels and most of the food particles actively pass across the villi walls and into the bloodstream. Some, like vitamin B_{12}, must be aided across by special proteins or other chemicals.

Blood that leaves the small intestine does not pass directly back to the heart, but first flows to the liver. Here fats, fat-soluble vitamins and other nutrients are stored, and some harmful chemicals absorbed with the food are deactivated.

The final stop for what remains of the food is the large intestine, or colon, where water and vitamins made by bacteria that live in the bowel are absorbed before the waste is eliminated.

The materials that the body's chemical plant derives from food and takes up into the bloodstream are known as nutrients. The body needs a variety of nutrients to sustain itself, power its machinery and rebuild its tissues. Here is a guide to the nutrients the body must derive from food:

Carbon

The element carbon is not itself a nutrient, but is part of many nutrients. Making up 45 percent of the body's dry weight (its weight minus the weight of water), carbon forms the backbone of organic molecules, such as proteins, fats and carbohydrates. In fact, the complex structures of many of these molecules, sometimes involving thousands of atoms, are made possible by the special properties of the carbon atom.

Among these properties is the ability to form four bonds or links with other atoms, including other carbon atoms. Carbon atoms can link with one another and with other atoms to form long chains, rings, helices and other configurations. These shapes, and the other atoms linked to the carbon atoms, give organic molecules their unique properties. Organic molecules, that is, chemicals with at least one carbon atom, come in a wide variety of sizes, ranging from methane, which has only one carbon atom and four hydrogen atoms, to myosin, a protein in muscle tissue that consists of well over 200,000 atoms.

Water

Life most likely began in water and life on earth cannot survive without it. If you doubt that water is important to human beings, consider this: About 60 percent of the weight of the human body is water. Water accounts for 80 percent of the weight of a typical cell. Of every 100 molecules in the body, 99 are water molecules.

A simple molecule (one oxygen atom bound to two hydrogens, or H_2O), water is a truly amazing chemical. It can dissolve a wide range of substances, so it is an excellent medium for transporting food and oxygen to the body's cells. Chemical reactions tend to occur more readily in water, so it is the perfect host for the body's essential chemical interactions. Water also helps maintain a normal body temperature, is essential for the normal digestion of food and is involved in virtually every other bodily function.

Proteins and Amino Acids

The Greek word *proteios,* from which comes protein, means "of the first rank" and proteins do indeed occupy a high place in the chemistry of living things. Proteins are the workhorses among biological molecules. They make up most of the body's architecture. The cell membrane, for example, is partly protein, as are most of the cell's organelles. Muscle tendon, ligaments, skin, hair and connective tissue are all largely protein.

But the role of protein is not limited to structure. Hormones and enzymes are proteins, as is hemoglobin, the protein in red blood cells, which transports oxygen from the lungs to the body's tissues. Proteins clot blood, heal wounds, maintain the body's water and chemical balance and form the framework for the minerals that make bones and teeth strong.

In the digestive tract, proteins are broken down into amino acids, the subunits that link to form the long protein chains. There are 22 amino acids required for normal metabolism and growth. The body can make all but 9 of them. These 9, known as the essential amino acids, must be obtained from food. Most animal protein contains all 9 essential amino acids. Vegetable proteins are usually missing one or more of the 9, so vegetarians have to combine different types of vegetable protein daily.

Carbohydrates

All living things require energy, and carbohydrates provide the bulk of it. Composed of carbon, hydrogen and oxygen, carbohydrates can be broken down by cells into water and carbon dioxide to yield energy.

The simplest carbohydrates are known as sugars. Simple rings formed by five or six carbon atoms, sugars are found primarily in fruits and vegetables. The most important sugar for people is glucose, or blood sugar. Glucose is readily absorbed by cells and converted to energy. Sucrose, or table sugar, is a combination of one glucose molecule and one molecule of fructose, a sugar found in many fruits. Other types of sugars commonly found in food are lactose, a sugar found in milk, and dextrose, or corn sugar, which is found in many plants.

Simple sugars can be linked to form more complex sugars, like sucrose, and much larger molecules. These large carbohydrates, made up of thousands of sugar molecules, serve as storage vehicles for simple sugars in plants and animals. For example, starch is a complex carbohydrate made up of many molecules of glucose and is used for energy storage in plants. Glucose is stored as the carbohydrate glycogen in animals. In plants complex carbohydrates like cellulose are also used for structure and support.

Fats

Scientists call these nutrients lipids. All lipids share one characteristic: they are insoluble in water. From motor oil to cholesterol, water and lipids do not mix. Most lipids are made primarily of the elements carbon and hydrogen, a characteristic related to their insolubility in water.

There are three types of lipids in the human body: neutral fats, phospholipids and steroids. Phospholipids are components of the cell membrane. Steroids, such as cholesterol, are the basis of some of the body's hormones, including the male and female sex hormones. What we usually call fats (and this includes most of the lipids in our bodies) are actually neutral fats.

Depending on how they are organized, neutral fats are considered to be saturated or unsaturated. There is a large body of evidence that links consumption of diets high in saturated animal fats with atherosclerosis and coronary heart disease. As you will see in Chapter 9, there may be a link between unsaturated fats and cancer.

The primary function of neutral fats is energy storage. Excess calories are ultimately converted to fat, which is stored in the liver and in fatty deposits in various parts of the body. When one's food intake drops, for example when one goes on a diet, neutral fat reserves are called on to provide energy for the body.

Vitamins

Probably no class of nutrient is more widely misunderstood than vitamins. Bombarded by outrageous claims, glowing recommendations by health gurus and pet theories by scientists and nonscientists alike, the average American has become confused. Few people seem to know just what vitamins are and how much we need to consume.

Vitamins are not miracle cures, quick energy, aphrodisiacs or prolongers of life. Vitamins are organic molecules that are necessary in *very small amounts* for normal health and growth. They were discovered around the turn of the century when scientists noticed that a diet with adequate macronutrients—proteins, carbohydrates and fats—was not enough to sustain life. A biologist named Funk in 1912 called these compounds vitamins because he believed they belong to a class of molecules known as amines (as it turns out, some are amines and some are not). *Vita* is a Latin word meaning *life,* so vitamin really means "life-giving amine."

The functions and dietary sources of vitamins were often dis-

Table 1

Recommended Daily Dietary Allowances (RDAs)

	Age (years)	Weight (lbs)	Protein (g)	Fat-Soluble Vitamins			Water-Soluble Vitamins							Minerals					
				Vitamin A (μg R.E.)[a]	Vitamin D (μg)	Vitamin E (mg)	Vitamin C (mg)	Thiamin (mg)	Riboflavin (mg)	Niacin (mg)	Vitamin B6 (mg)	Folacin (μg)	Vitamin B12 (μg)	Calcium (mg)	Phosphorus (mg)	Magnesium (mg)	Iron (mg)	Zinc (mg)	Iodine (μg)
Infants	0-6 mo.	13	lb × 1 [b]	420	10	3	35	0.3	0.4	6	0.3	30	0.5	360	240	50	10	3	40
	6 mo.-1	20	lb × 0.9 [b]	400	10	4	35	0.5	0.6	8	0.6	45	1.5	540	360	70	15	5	50
Children	1-3	29	23	400	10	5	45	0.7	0.8	9	0.9	100	2.0	800	800	150	15	10	70
	4-6	44	30	500	10	6	45	0.9	1.0	11	1.3	200	2.5	800	800	200	10	10	90
	7-10	62	34	700	10	7	45	1.2	1.4	16	1.6	300	3.0	800	800	250	10	10	120
Males	11-14	99	45	1000	10	8	50	1.4	1.6	18	1.8	400	3.0	1200	1200	350	18	15	150
	15-18	145	56	1000	10	10	60	1.4	1.7	18	2.0	400	3.0	1200	1200	400	18	15	150
	19-22	154	56	1000	7.5	10	60	1.5	1.7	19	2.2	400	3.0	800	800	350	10	15	150
	23-50	154	56	1000	5	10	60	1.4	1.6	18	2.2	400	3.0	800	800	350	10	15	150
	51+	154	56	1000	5	10	60	1.2	1.4	16	2.2	400	3.0	800	800	350	10	15	150
Females	11-14	101	46	800	10	8	50	1.1	1.3	15	1.8	400	3.0	1200	1200	300	18	15	150
	15-18	120	46	800	10	8	60	1.1	1.3	14	2.0	400	3.0	1200	1200	300	18	15	150
	19-22	120	44	800	7.5	8	60	1.1	1.3	14	2.0	400	3.0	800	800	300	18	15	150
	23-50	120	44	800	5	8	60	1.0	1.2	13	2.0	400	3.0	800	800	300	18	15	150
	51+	120	44	800	5	8	60	1.0	1.2	13	2.0	400	3.0	800	800	300	10	15	150
Pregnant[c]			+30	+200	+5	+2	+20	+0.4	+0.3	+2	+0.6	+400	+1.0	+400	+400	+150	d	+5	+25
Nursing[c]			+20	+400	+5	+3	+40	+0.5	+0.5	+5	+0.5	+100	+1.0	+400	+400	+150	d	+10	+50

a Retinol equivalents. 1 retinol equivalent = 1 μg retinol or 6 μg β-carotene.

b Multiply body weight of infant times number shown to get daily protein requirement in grams.

c The figures in these rows preceded by the "+" sign indicate the additional requirements, above the RDA, for these nutrients during pregnancy and breast feeding.

d The increased requirement during pregnancy cannot be met by the iron content of typical American diets nor by existing iron stores; therefore the use of 30–60 mg of supplemental iron is recommended. Iron needs while nursing are not substantially different from those of nonpregnant women, but continued supplementation for 2–3 months after delivery is advisable in order to replenish stores depleted by pregnancy.

Estimated Safe and Adequate Daily Dietary Intakes of Selected Vitamins and Minerals[a]

	Age (years)	Vitamins			Trace Minerals[b]						Macrominerals		
		Vitamin K (µg)	Biotin (µg)	Pantothenic Acid (mg)	Copper (mg)	Manganese (mg)	Fluoride (mg)	Chromium (mg)	Selenium (mg)	Molybdenum (mg)	Sodium (mg)	Potassium (mg)	Chloride (mg)
Infants	0-6 mo.	12	35	2	0.5-0.7	0.5-0.7	0.1-0.5	0.01-0.04	0.01-0.04	0.03-0.06	115-350	350-925	275-700
	6 mo.-1	10-20	50	3	0.7-1.0	0.7-1.0	0.2-1.0	0.02-0.06	0.02-0.06	0.04-0.08	250-750	425-1275	400-1200
Children	1-3	15-30	65	3	1.0-1.5	1.0-1.5	0.5-1.5	0.02-0.08	0.02-0.08	0.05-0.1	325-975	550-1650	500-1500
	4-6	20-40	85	3-4	1.5-2.0	1.5-2.0	1.0-2.5	0.03-0.12	0.03-0.12	0.06-0.15	450-1350	775-2325	700-1200
	7-10	30-60	120	4-5	2.0-2.5	2.0-3.0	1.5-2.5	0.05-0.2	0.05-0.2	0.1 -0.3	600-1800	1000-3000	925-2775
	11+	50-100	100-200	4-7	2.0-3.0	2.5-5.0	1.5-2.5	0.05-0.2	0.05-0.2	0.15-0.5	900-2700	1525-4575	1400-4200
Adults		70-140	100-200	4-7	2.0-3.0	2.5-5.0	1.5-4.0	0.05-0.2	0.05-0.2	0.15-0.5	1100-3300	1875-5625	1700-5100

a Because there is less information on which to base allowances, these figures are not given in the RDA table, but are provided here in the form of ranges of recommended intakes.

b Since the toxic levels for many trace elements may be only several times usual intakes, the upper levels for the trace elements given in this table should not be habitually exceeded.

The Recommended Daily Dietary Allowances and the Estimated Safe and Adequate Daily Dietary Intakes are established by the Food and Nutrition Board of the National Academy of Sciences-National Research Council. The figures in these tables were revised in 1980. They are intended to provide adequate nutrition for most normal people in the U.S. under normal environmental stresses.

covered before their chemical structures, so they were identified by letters, a practice that we continue today. There are 13 compounds generally agreed to be vitamins and a few others either tentatively or erroneously given this designation. As you will see, vitamins perform many jobs in the body, but most of them are co-enzymes, which means they aid enzymes in catalyzing biochemical reactions.

Unlike the larger organic nutrients, which are broken down and consumed in the course of normal metabolism, vitamins generally are not dismantled and can be used over and over by the body. This is why only small amounts must be consumed to replace those that are destroyed or lost in the urine or feces.

Four of the vitamins, A, D, E and K, are soluble in fat. They must be linked with fats or bile in the digestive tract before they can be absorbed through the intestinal wall. Because they are stored in body fat, they are not excreted readily and do not have to be replaced as often as the water-soluble vitamins. But they can also build up to large and sometimes toxic levels if consumed in excessive quantities for prolonged periods. This is especially true of vitamin A.

The remaining vitamins, eight Bs and C, are soluble in water. They are not readily stored in the body and are lost in the urine, so they must be consumed in adequate amounts every day. Table 1 lists the current recommended dietary allowances of all 13 vitamins.

The best sources of vitamins are plants. Bacteria in our intestines also make some of the vitamins we need, although not enough to sustain life. Liver is an excellent source of the fat-soluble vitamins, because this is where many are stored in animal bodies. However, the liver is also where the body stores many pollutants. Consequently, liver should not be relied upon as a primary source of vitamins.

Here is a beginner's guide to the vitamins:

VITAMIN A: When you were growing up, your mother may have told you that yellow and orange vegetables, like carrots, were good for your eyes. She was right. These vegetables contain vitamin A. Vitamin A is the basis of the visual pigments that allow you to see. In the retina of your eyes, there are two types of receptors, specialized cells that respond to light. Cones respond to the primary colors of light—red, blue and green—while rods detect dim light. The light-sensitive pigments in all of these cells are derived from vitamin A.

Vitamin A also promotes the normal growth of a class of cells known as epithelium, which includes the skin, hair, mucous membranes and the lining of the lungs, digestive tract, urogenital system and other organs. One sign of a vitamin A deficiency is the hardening and roughening of the skin, caused by the abnormal growth of the skin epithelium. As you will see in Chapter 6, cancer of the skin and other epithelium may be promoted by a lack of adequate vitamin A.

Also required for normal bone growth, reproduction, tooth development and resistance to bacteria, vitamin A is fat-soluble and is stored in the liver and other fatty areas. It comes naturally in two forms—retinol and carotene. Carotene, the form found in plants, is split in the intestine into two molecules of retinol, the form used by the body.

In addition to yellow, orange and dark green vegetables, vitamin A is found in liver, cheese, milk, eggs, butter and fortified margarine. A deficiency of vitamin A is characterized by night blindness, roughened and dry skin, impaired bone growth, increased susceptibility to infections and reduced functioning of the gastrointestinal, genitourinary and respiratory systems. Very high doses of retinol can be quite toxic, so megadoses of this type of vitamin A should not be taken. Too much retinol can cause headaches, blurred vision, nausea, diarrhea, loss of appetite, dry skin, liver and kidney damage, an excessive amount of calcium in the blood, fatigue, hair loss and brain damage. Excess retinol has also caused birth defects in animal studies. With the exception of a yellowish tinge to the skin that sometimes develops, large amounts of carotene are not known to cause adverse reactions.

THE B VITAMINS: In the late 1800s, it was observed that hens fed mostly polished rice (rice that has been milled) developed inflammation of the nerves similar to beriberi, a deficiency disease of humans. When a diet of brown rice was substituted, the symptoms disappeared. It was not until 1926 that a factor was isolated that accounted for the antiberiberi effect of the unpolished rice. It was called vitamin B, a name later changed to B_1 and B_2 after it was found that there were two vitamins in the rice hull, one that prevented beriberi and another that was necessary for growth. Subsequently, B_2 turned out to be not one substance but several. These are the members of the B vitamin family, a family that includes the original B_1, which is now called thiamine.

Though they differ in structure, all the B vitamins play a similar role in the body—helping enzymes do their job. Enzymes speed the progress of biological reactions, without being altered themselves. They generally consist of a protein portion and another chemical called a cofactor. The cofactor can be a number of minerals, including copper, cobalt, magnesium and zinc, or a vitamin, or both. Many of the B vitamins are cofactors of the enzymes that help cells utilize food.

B_1 OR THIAMINE: This vitamin helps cells use carbohydrates by acting as a cofactor for 24 enzymes. It is also necessary for the production of acetylcholine, a chemical involved in the process by which impulses are transmitted between nerve cells. B_1 is found in whole-wheat grains, wheat germ, liver and kidney, pork, peas, peanuts, beans, nuts, oranges and many other fruits and vegetables. This nutrient is also manufactured by intestinal bacteria.

Too little thiamine in the diet can cause beriberi, which is characterized by partial paralysis of the skeletal muscles and the smooth muscles of the digestive tract. This can result in atrophying of the limbs and digestive disturbances, such as colitis, constipation and diarrhea. Another symptom of a thiamine deficiency is polyneuritis, which can impair the spatial sense and the sense of touch and can also result in the stunting of growth in children. No specific symptoms of excessive doses or megadoses of thiamine are known.

B_2, OR RIBOFLAVIN: Found in yeast, kidney, liver, beef, veal, lamb, eggs, whole-wheat products, asparagus, peas, beets, peanuts, dark green vegetables, mushrooms and enriched processed foods, riboflavin is a cofactor in enzymes that allow cells to use carbohydrates, proteins and fats and is also necessary for normal growth. A deficiency of riboflavin can result in cracks in the skin, especially in the corners of the mouth, and dermatitis. Blurred vision, cataracts, ulcers of the cornea and anemia have also been seen. There appear to be no effects from taking excessive doses.

NIACIN, OR B_3, NICOTINAMIDE, AND NICOTINIC ACID: An essential component of enzymes involved in the production of energy in cells, niacin also assists in the breakdown of fats. Niacin is found in lean meat, fish, liver, yeast, whole-grain breads and cereals, peas, beans, nuts and eggs. The amino acid tryptophan can be converted by the body to niacin with the aid of other B vitamins. Too little niacin causes pellagra, a disorder characterized by inflamed skin, diarrhea, confusion, irritability and swelling of the tongue. Too much niacin may cause duodenal ulcers, low blood sugar and other disorders.

B_6, OR PYRIDOXINE, PYRIDOXAL OR PYRIDOXAMINE: This vitamin helps the body make and utilize protein; break down fat; make red blood cells; produce antibodies; and synthesize such compounds as serotonin, which constricts blood vessels and helps us sleep. Formed by bacteria in the gut, B_6 is also found in whole-grain cereals and bread, tomatoes, yellow corn, spinach, green beans, bananas, poultry, fish, liver and yogurt. Dermatitis and cracks at the corners of the mouth, nausea, dizziness, depression and convulsions may result from a deficiency, while no effects from high doses are known.

PANTOTHENIC ACID: This vitamin, which is essential for the normal utilization of carbohydrates, proteins and fats by cells, is also involved in the production of hormones. It is found in liver, kidney, dark green vegetables, cereals, yeast, eggs and dried legumes. It is stored in the liver and kidneys, so a daily intake is not necessary. Deficiencies have only been created in humans experimentally. An excess of pantothenic acid may cause an increased need for thiamine.

BIOTIN: Found in liver, kidney, egg yolks, yeast, dark green vegetables and green beans, biotin is also manufactured by bacteria in the gastrointestinal tract. Although egg yolks contain biotin, raw egg white (in eggnog, for example) will destroy it. This vitamin is required for the normal use of carbohydrates, proteins and fats by cells. Although not usually seen, a biotin deficiency causes depression, fatigue, muscle pain and nausea. There are no known negative effects of megadoses.

FOLACIN, OR FOLIC ACID: Essential for the formation of normal red and white blood cells, folic acid also helps create some of the components of the DNA molecule. Liver, kidneys, green leafy vegetables and dried legumes are all sources of this vitamin, which is also synthesized by intestinal bacteria. Too little folic acid may result in megaloblastic anemia, an anemia characterized by abnormally large red blood cells. A deficiency during pregnancy can cause spontaneous abortions or birth defects. No effects of excessive doses are known.

B_{12} OR CYANOCOBALAMIN: Vitamin B_{12} is essential for the normal development of red blood cells. The red cells will mature into functioning carriers of oxygen only in the presence of this compound. B_{12} also helps nerve cells in the central nervous system derive energy from carbohydrates.

Vitamin B_{12} is in liver, meat, kidney, milk, cheese and eggs, but is the only B vitamin not found in any vegetables. Strict vegetarians should take a B_{12} supplement to avoid the risk of pernicious anemia. Characterized by weakness, a sore tongue, tingling and numbness of the extremities, nausea, vomiting and diarrhea, pernicious anemia is usually treated by intramuscular injections of vitamin B_{12}.

Vegetarians are not the only ones at risk to developing pernicious anemia. A substance known as intrinsic factor must be present in the digestive tract before vitamin B_{12}, a large molecule, can be absorbed through the intestinal wall. Secreted by the stomach lining, intrinsic factor seems to pull B_{12} through the intestine. Those who have stopped producing an adequate amount of intrinsic factor (which occasionally happens after the age of 40), or who have had a portion of their stomach removed, will not absorb adequate amounts of B_{12}.

VITAMIN C, OR ASCORBIC ACID: In the evolution of certain mammals, including humans, nature seems to have played an unfortunate trick. All mammals, with the exception of humans, other primates, bats and guinea pigs, make their own vitamin C. Your pet dog or cat will never need to eat fruits and vegetables, but you must, every day. How this evolutionary quirk came about, scientists are not sure, but the roles vitamin C plays in the body have become much clearer over the years.

This water-soluble vitamin is abundant in most fruits and vegetables, especially citrus fruits, tomatoes, potatoes, green peppers, and dark green vegetables. It plays an important role in the formation and healing of many tissues, including collagen, the key ingredient of connective tissue. Found in bone, skin, ligaments and cartilage, connective tissue helps the lungs stretch as we breathe, holds our organs together and helps us move about.

Vitamin C also enhances the activity of certain enzymes, helps the body absorb iron, assures that blood will clot when necessary and aids in the healing of wounds and bone fractures. When the body does not get enough vitamin C, the result is scurvy. Many of the symptoms of this disease stem from the impaired formation of connective tissue. The gums become swollen and bleed, wounds don't heal properly, joints become tender and muscles degenerate. Teeth may become loose and more susceptible to cavities as the body's resistance to infection diminishes. Anemia may also develop, and wounds may bleed excessively or bruises develop too easily.

The consequences of taking large doses of vitamin C are more controversial, if only because of the number of people who tout vitamin C megadoses as sure cures for everything from the common cold to cancer. To date, little evidence supports these claims, while some evidence suggests that vitamin C can cause health problems in a small percentage of the population when taken in massive doses. While the body needs only 30 to 60 milligrams of vitamin C each day, some nutritional therapies call for doses as high as several grams.

Very large amounts of vitamin C can precipitate the formation of kidney and bladder stones in people who are at risk and cause diarrhea, urinary tract irritations and other symptoms. In addition, the body seems to gradually adapt to the higher doses, actually requiring them to maintain health. When a megadoser returns to a normal intake, there is a risk of developing scurvy until the body readjusts. This can be particularly dangerous in infants born to women who take megadoses during pregnancy.

Despite these effects, there seem to be benefits from taking doses of vitamin C greater than what is needed to fend off scurvy. For example, a team of researchers found that the daily dose that could prevent scurvy in guinea pigs did nothing to combat the toxic effects of a pesticide known as dieldrin. However, guinea pigs that received a dose eight times greater were able to break down the pesticide nearly twice as fast as test animals that received a normal dose. Another researcher found that four grams of vitamin C per day reduced by 70 percent the quantity of a cancer-causing substance known as nitrosamine in human feces. A study in the Soviet Union showed that a dose of 100 milligrams per day could aid in eliminating excess fluoride from the bodies of industrial workers.

The results of these and other studies have led some scientists to argue that the current recommended daily allowance for vitamin C is too low. In fact, one researcher, noting that many animals synthesize huge amounts of vitamin C when under stress, argued that anyone who does not take 10 to 20 grams of vitamin C a day is suffering from low-level scurvy.

VITAMIN D: Some have argued that vitamin D is not really a vitamin at all. Under ideal conditions, the ultraviolet rays of sunlight striking the skin will convert a compound called provitamin D_3, a derivative of cholesterol, into vitamin D. Theoretically, the skin of Caucasians can produce all of the vitamin D they need. In reality, because most Americans live in higher latitudes where the sun is less intense and where clothes cover most of the skin a great deal of the time, the average person must take in vitamin D in the diet.

Vitamin D plays a vitally important role in the intestinal absorption of calcium, a component of bones and teeth. The absorption of calcium takes place at a much faster pace when vitamin D is present. In addition, vitamin D is important for the normal growth and development of bones. When vitamin D is lacking, the bones fail to incorporate calcium and phosphorus and become brittle and weak.

This condition is known as rickets when it occurs in children and osteomalacia in adults. Rickets results when bones do not get enough calcium as they develop and become misshapen. Legs bow and growth is stunted. The head can grow large and square and the skull bones become so soft they may crack like parchment. In addition, the liver and spleen may become enlarged, making the abdomen protrude. Osteomalacia, the adult form of rickets, is marked by soft and brittle bones that may become deformed. This is usually accompanied by pains in the extremities.

Both forms of rickets are reversible with treatment, usually involving large doses of vitamin D.

There is a danger, however, in prescribing too high a dose, as vitamin D has serious health effects in very high concentrations. Nausea, loss of appetite, high blood pressure, excessive urine excretion, excessive thirst and kidney stones are some of the consequences. In addition, the soft tissues throughout the body, such as the heart, lungs, kidneys and joints, may develop calcium deposits and, ironically, the bones may become fragile.

Vitamin D is found in egg yolks, butter, fortified milk, liver, fish liver oils, tuna, salmon, herring, sardines and oysters.

VITAMIN E: More hopeful claims are made about this vitamin than about almost any other food constituent. It has been said that vitamin E may prevent muscular dystrophy, enhance sexual endurance, prevent heart disease, improve the health of people who have heart problems, increase one's athletic abilities and prevent or slow the aging process.

There are several functions of vitamin E that scientists are certain of. Many systems in the body, in particular cell membranes, have lipids that are destroyed when they react with free oxygen as well as ozone and other air pollutants. Vitamin E is an antioxidant, which means that it protects these lipids from reacting with oxygen. It is also known to protect vitamin A from the same fate.

Vitamin E may affect the enzymes involved in the formation of red blood cells, aiding the production of these oxygen carriers. This vitamin may also be involved in the formation of DNA and may protect the liver from toxic chemicals.

Although such symptoms as reproductive failure and muscular dystrophy appear in laboratory animals deprived of vitamin E, deficiencies are almost never seen in humans and complications from overdoses of this vitamin are not generally reported. Vitamin E is found in lettuce and other leafy green vegetables, fresh nuts, wheat germ, vegetable and seed oils, whole grains, dried beans and liver.

VITAMIN K: Manufactured in substantial quantities by intestinal bacteria, vitamin K is also found in spinach, cauliflower, cabbage, peas, potatoes, cereals and liver. The K in vitamin K stands for the German word for coagulation, and in fact this vitamin is essential for normal blood clotting. Vitamin K helps the liver produce prothrombin, a chemical involved in the multistep clotting process. A deficiency of vitamin K can cause hemorrhaging, especially in infants. An excess has been known to cause jaundice in children.

Minerals

Like vitamins, minerals are needed in relatively small amounts to sustain growth and health. But, while vitamins are biological molecules, minerals are inorganic, that is, without a carbon atom. Minerals are generally divided into two classes: the macrominerals, which are needed in small quantities, and the trace minerals, which are needed in very small or trace amounts.

Most minerals are components of enzymes and help regulate body processes. Others make up part of the body's structure, for example calcium and phosphorus, which give strength to bones and teeth. And one mineral, iron, is an important part of the protein hemoglobin, which allows red blood cells to transport oxygen.

As with vitamins, an absence of minerals can cause a variety of deficiency symptoms. Also like vitamins, minerals can cause serious health problems if taken in excessively large doses, something that an unfortunate number of enthusiasts who attempt to promote good health with megadoses of minerals are finding out.

Here is an introduction to some of the more important minerals. Table 2 describes additional essential minerals. Below and in the table, *macro* means macromineral and *trace,* trace mineral. The RDAs for many of the minerals can be found in Table 1.

CALCIUM (MACRO): This mineral makes up about 2 percent of the weight of an average body. That is about 2 pounds of calcium for a 100-pound person. Most of that—about 99 percent—is found in bones and teeth, where it lends rigidity and support. Calcium helps muscles contract and impulses propagate along nerve fibers and is also important for the maintenance of cell membranes. Normal blood clotting and the absorption of vitamin B_{12} by the digestive tract depend on calcium. The body must have vitamin D to absorb calcium (see vitamin D above). Vitamin C, the milk sugar lactose, and exercise also help the body assimilate calcium. Too much protein or fat and too much phosphorus, though, increase the body's need for calcium. The best source of calcium is milk, which contains about 300 milligrams—about a third of the daily requirement for a young adult and half of a child's daily need—per cup. Green leafy vegetables (such as spinach, kale and collard greens), yogurt, dried beans and citrus fruits are also good sources.

When the body does not get enough calcium from food it begins to draw on its store in the bones to provide enough for nerve and muscle activity. If the deficiency is serious, the bones may weaken, leading to rickets in children and osteomalacia in adults (see vitamin D above). Megadoses of calcium can cause calcium deposits in the soft tissues of the body. Too much calcium can also cause lethargy and impair the absorption of iron, manganese, zinc and other essential minerals.

To derive the benefits attributed to excess calcium, or simply to insure an adequate intake of this mineral, some people have taken to using bone meal supplements. This is a dangerous practice. Bones are the natural repositories of many minerals, including harmful ones like lead and strontium. There have, in fact, been cases of lead poisoning resulting from eating bone meal. This is a particularly dangerous practice for pregnant women, since lead is known to cause birth defects.

COPPER (TRACE): This element is required for the manufacture of red blood cells. Copper, which helps the body store iron, is a component of several enzymes in the respiratory system and is also part of the enzyme that helps make melanin, the pigment in skin.

Most unprocessed foods are good sources of copper, but organ meats, fish, nuts, oysters, dried peas and beans, eggs, spinach, asparagus and whole-wheat flour are especially rich sources. A deficiency of copper can cause anemia, weakness, impaired growth and development, abnormal development of the lungs and poor utilization of iron by the body. Too much copper can precipitate vomiting and diarrhea and pain in the stomach and esophagus. Because acid foods can leach copper out of copper pots, it is not wise to use unlined copper pots for cooking.

TABLE **2** | **OTHER MINERALS REQUIRED BY THE BODY**

Mineral/Source	Functions
Chloride (macro)/table salt, sea salt	Helps regulate the balance of acids and bases in the blood and maintain the body's water balance. Part of hydrochloric acid made by stomach.
Chromium (trace)/whole grain cereals, liver, dried brewer's yeast, cheese	Along with insulin, it helps the body derive energy from glucose.
Cobalt (trace)/meat, eggs, dairy products	This mineral is important because it is a part of vitamin B_{12}.
Fluoride (trace)/fish, tea, fluoridated water	Contributes to the development of strong teeth and bones.
Iodine (macro)/seafood, seaweed, sea salt, iodized salt	Component of thyroid hormones that control the body's metabolic rate.
Potassium (macro)/orange juice, bananas, dried fruit, meat, peanut butter, potatoes, coffee, tea, cocoa	Required for normal muscle contraction and nerve activity. Helps regulate the balance of body fluids and acid/base balance in body.
Sodium (macro)/table salt, meat, fish, poultry, eggs, milk, processed foods	This mineral controls the body's water balance, controlling the flow of water in and out of cells and protecting the body from dehydration. It also acts with calcium to maintain normal heart action.
Sulfur (macro)/beef, wheat germ, peanuts, dried beans	Found in sulfur-containing amino acids, it is part of proteins in hair, skin and nails; also part of insulin and the B vitamins biotin and thiamine.

Consequences of a Deficiency	Results of an Excess
Quite rare.	Disruption of blood acid/base balance.
Symptoms similar to diabetes.	Bad taste in the mouth, cramps, diarrhea.
Causes anemia similar to that of a vitamin B_{12} deficiency in animals; symptoms unusual in people, but can occur in vegetarians, since plants have only trace amounts of cobalt.	An overdose in children can be fatal; in adults, it can cause a loss of appetite, nausea, vomiting, deafness and excessive growth of the thyroid gland.
Excess cavities; possibly brittle bones in the elderly.	Mottling of the teeth; excessive doses can cause damage to the bones.
Goiter, which is characterized by an enlarged thyroid and low production of the thyroid hormones. In infants, can cause cretinism—arrested physical and mental development, anemia, protruding abdomen, swollen tongue, puffy face and hands, loss of hair and sensitivity to cold.	Rare. When iodine poisoning occurs, includes brown stains on lips and mouth, vomiting and bloody diarrhea.
Muscle weakness, dizziness, excessive thirst, mental confusion and kidney and lung failure.	Paralysis and irregular heartbeat.
Because of the amount of salt (sodium chloride) Americans eat, a deficiency is virtually unknown.	It is believed that excess sodium, from food or from drinking water contaminated by road salt, may be a contributor to the development of high blood pressure.
Inflammation of skin and imperfect development of hair and nails.	Unknown.

IRON (MACRO): Iron is found in two complex molecules (called pigments) that serve as carriers for oxygen in the body. The first is hemoglobin. A component of red blood cells, it carries oxygen from the lungs to all of the tissues of the body. The second is myoglobin, a similar protein, which acts as a storehouse in skeletal muscles, holding on to a supply of oxygen until the muscle is called on to do strenuous work. Iron is also part of certain enzymes, including one that helps the body store energy.

A deficiency of iron results in anemia, the shortness of breath, tiredness and pallor caused by failure to get enough oxygen to the cells. Too much iron in the diet can cause a toxic accumulation of the mineral in the heart and other organs.

MAGNESIUM (MACRO): Magnesium activates the enzymes that are involved in the storage of energy in the body. It also helps the body adjust to cold, allows nerve impulses to travel to skeletal muscles and aids in the contraction of those muscles. It is a component of bones and is essential for the manufacture of proteins.

Found in bananas, whole-grain products, dried beans, milk, nuts, dark green leafy vegetables and seeds, magnesium can interfere with the functions of the nervous system if present in large amounts. A deficiency causes muscle spasms, twitches, cramps, weakness, depression, insomnia and irregular heartbeat.

PHOSPHORUS (MACRO): If importance is gauged by the number of functions a nutrient performs, then phosphorus may well be the most important of the minerals. A component of DNA, the molecule of heredity, phosphorus is also essential for normal muscle contraction and nerve activity. It makes up a portion of normal bones and teeth, where 80 percent of the body's phosphorus is found.

Phosphorus is part of the structure of many enzymes and is involved in the transport and storage of energy throughout the body. It is also part of a buffer system that helps keep the blood from becoming too acid or basic. Meat, poultry, fish, eggs, dairy products, nuts and dried peas and beans are all good sources of phosphorus.

Deficiencies of phosphorus are rare and are sometimes caused by the overuse of antacids. Weakness, fatigue and bone pain are the symptoms. Too much phosphorus can precipitate a calcium deficiency.

SELENIUM (TRACE): Found in varying amounts in seafood, meat, whole grain cereals, poultry and egg yolks, selenium's role in the body seems to be similar to that of vitamin E. Like vitamin E, selenium is an antioxidant and acts to protect the lipids in cell membranes from destruction by free oxygen and certain air pollutants.

Vitamin E and selenium can interact in protecting cell membranes and, in fact, selenium can perform some of the functions of vitamin E in an animal deficient in this vitamin. In some studies the amount of selenium needed has been found to be inversely related to the amount of vitamin E in the diet. In addition to protecting membranes, selenium is an integral part of several proteins and enzymes, particularly those involved in the transfer and storage of energy in the body. Selenium also protects the liver, especially in the case of a vitamin E deficiency.

Selenium deficiency is unknown in humans. Exposure to too much selenium (something that rarely occurs in people, but that can be a danger in areas where drinking water wells pass through shale rich in soluble selenium) has produced depression, nervousness, skin irritations, stomach disorders and a garlic odor of the breath and sweat. Some studies have concluded that high levels of selenium exposure can cause cavities and cancer. However, serious experimental flaws mar these studies. In fact, work with animals indicates that selenium may actually prevent cancer. When mice were treated with an agent that caused skin cancers and then exposed to a cancer-promoting compound mixed with selenium, their incidence of cancer was markedly lower than that of animals that were exposed just to the promoter. Other studies have shown a relationship between the level of selenium in the soil and plant life in various areas of the country and the rates of several types of cancers, with the cancer rate significantly higher in areas with low selenium.

ZINC (MACRO): This mineral is a component of as many as 100 enzymes in the body. It is involved in normal wound healing and is required for growth and development. The requirement for zinc seems to be linked to the level of iron and copper in the diet.

Zinc is found in many foods, especially beef, eggs, liver, poultry, seafood, whole grains, peas, carrots and pure maple syrup. A deficiency of zinc can lead to loss of appetite, impaired sense of taste, slow healing of wounds and diminished growth and development in children. Zinc poisoning is not common, although it does occasionally occur in people who drink water from galvanized pipes for long periods of time. The symptoms include loss of appetite, muscle stiffness and pain, anemia and nausea.

CHAPTER 4

The Chemistry of Disease:
Toxicology and Epidemiology

Just as it is chemical elements and compounds that drive the processes of life, it is chemical intruders that can make us sick and even kill us. These chemical villains run the gamut from essential substances, such as vitamins or medications, which we may consume to excess, to potent poisons that can kill with just a speck or a mere drop.

This chapter explores the sciences of poisons and disease, toxicology and epidemiology. We will look at what constitutes a poison, how harmful substances make us sick, how the body deactivates some poisons and makes others more poisonous and how certain chemicals cause mutations, birth defects and cancer. We will also look at the tests scientists use to study poisons and at how animals and human subjects are used to predict the effects of toxic and carcinogenic substances on the human body.

It is difficult to fully appreciate how nutrition can alter the effects of poisons on the human body without first understanding what those effects are. For example, in later chapters we will look at the ways in which it is thought certain vitamins and minerals reduce the body's chances of developing cancer. But before reading these sections, it would be helpful to understand how cancers arise in the first place. We will also in later chapters talk extensively about scientific studies that have been conducted to probe the interaction between nutrients and toxic chemicals. Thus we have also included in this chapter brief introductions to the laboratory and field tests most often used by toxicologists, epidemiologists and other public health scientists.

POISONS: HOW THEY WORK

Whether a particular substance will harm the body depends on a number of factors, including the route of entry. For example, when asbestos is inhaled it can cause lung cancer. However, whether it causes cancer when ingested with drinking water remains to be definitively shown. Another factor is dose. A large amount of a particular compound, like cadmium, may have an immediate and serious effect on the body if ingested all at once. If the same amount of the compound is ingested over a long period of time, it may be relatively harmless.

Poisonous substances can have a wide variety of effects on the body, ranging from minor skin irritations to cancer. The effects are usually divided into local and whole-body—systemic—effects. One local effect is contact dermatitis, a skin condition very much like poison ivy that is caused by repeated contact with a variety of industrial chemicals. When inhaled, fumes and dust can burn or irritate the lining of the respiratory tract, another type of local reaction.

The majority of toxic effects are systemic. In these, the poisons enter the bloodstream and gain access to all parts of the body. Once in the body, the poisons may attack a specific organ, as the heavy metal cadmium attacks the kidneys and the organic solvent carbon tetrachloride damages the liver. Some poisons, like cyanide, assault cells and tissues in general.

Among the many ways poisons can damage the body are:

—By keeping the digestive tract from absorbing necessary nutrients or by preventing these nutrients from doing their jobs in the body. Toxins can also deplete the body's stores of nutrients or chemically alter nutrients so they are no longer effective. Pesticides, for example, deplete stores of vitamins A, D and E and nicotine can destroy vitamin C in the digestive tract before it can be absorbed.

—By interfering with the activity of enzymes, as lead and mercury do. In this way, toxins prevent or slow critical chemical reactions, halt the formation by the body of important compounds or allow unwanted chemicals to accumulate.

—By hampering life-sustaining processes. Carbon monoxide,

for example, prevents oxygen from binding to the hemoglobin in red blood cells.

—By damaging or destroying cell membranes. Ozone destroys fats in the membranes of the cells lining the respiratory tract.

—By blocking nerve impulses. The toxin produced by the botulism bacteria blocks the flow of impulses to the skeletal muscles and can cause paralysis.

—By harming the hereditary material in cells. Ultraviolet light, for example, can damage DNA, the molecule that contains the cell's genetic information.

—By preventing the cell from repairing its DNA, as caffeine does, and, therefore, increasing the risk of mutations, birth defects and cancer.

—By causing fatty lesions in the liver, reducing the effectiveness of this organ and possibly inducing cancer. The solvents chloroform and carbon tetrachloride fall into this category.

METABOLISM: HOW THE BODY CREATES AND DESTROYS POISONS

Before a chemical can cause a systemic reaction, it must enter the body. This means crossing one of the body's three main barriers—the skin, the lungs or the digestive tract. Upon entering the body, the pollutant or drug may act directly on the blood, as lead does, or it may travel to a specific tissue. Some chemicals are capable of causing tissue damage from the moment they enter the body to the moment they are removed as waste by the kidneys or another excretory organ. Others are stored temporarily and rather innocuously in bones or become bound to plasma proteins in the blood. They may be released from the bones or blood over a period of time and gradually reach target organs where they cause toxic reactions.

Chemicals, such as pesticides, that are stored in the body's fat may enter the bloodstream when the body utilizes those fats for energy. Chemicals tied up in the bones may be released into the blood if the bones begin to demineralize due to a vitamin D or calcium deficiency. A calcium deficiency and the resultant loss of calcium from bones is common during pregnancy, which suggests that pregnant women and the children they carry may be at higher than normal risk to heavy metals.

Most chemicals do not go unchallenged by the body. When they reach the liver, special enzymes may break them down or metabolize them into other, less toxic compounds. Cyanide, for example, is converted by the liver to a chemical known as thiocyanate, which is several hundred times less toxic than cyanide. While the liver disarms cyanide and many other toxins, it activates others by chemically changing them or splitting them into even more harmful substances. Methanol, a mildly poisonous alcohol, is converted to formaldehyde, a much more toxic compound, which is also believed to be a carcinogen. The common painkiller and sedative codeine is metabolized to the narcotic morphine. The rat poison fluoroacetate is toxic because liver enzymes convert it to fluorocitrate, a substance that is highly lethal to cells. In fact, the toxicity of many substances may be due not to the original or parent compounds, but to the compounds they are metabolized to in the body.

Some chemicals can trigger the immune system. They do this by acting as antigens and triggering the formation of antibodies. An antibody is a protein the body makes to fight off a specific bacterium, virus or chemical intruder. Once the body has produced these antibodies, subsequent exposure to the chemical will trigger an allergic response. Sometimes these allergic reactions can be quite serious. For example, the widely used antibiotic penicillin causes a reaction in about ten percent of the people who take it. The reaction ranges from skin rashes, hives and flulike symptoms to anaphylaxis, a severe and sometimes fatal type of allergic reaction.

CARCINOGENS: CHEMICALS THAT CAUSE CANCER

Several of the more serious effects of chemicals involve alteration or destruction of the cell's genetic repository. If a chemical causes a change in a gene (a section of a chromosome and a basic unit of heredity), the result is called a mutation. If the mutation occurs in a sex cell or in a critical cell in an embryo or fetus (altering an important structure or function), the result may be a birth defect, a genetic disorder, a spontaneous abortion or a stillbirth. When the mutation arises in the cells of a child or adult, the effect may range from no measurable change all the way to uncontrollable cell division, a condition called cancer.

The mechanisms by which a chemical converts a normal cell to a mutant and ultimately to a cancer cell are not fully understood. One theory, backed by a growing body of data, says that a mutagen or carcinogen (cancer-causing chemical) is likely to be a molecule that has a strong attraction for electrons, the tiny atomic particles that circle the nucleus or core of an atom. The nucleic acids and proteins that make up molecules of deoxyribonucleic acid (DNA, the molecule that stores genetic information) are rich in electrons. The electron-hungry carcinogens react with the electron-wealthy sections of DNA, removing electrons and causing irreversible change. One apparent problem with this theory is that many known carcinogens do not strongly attract electrons. It is now believed that this type of carcinogen must be transformed by the body (usually in the liver) to the ultimate, electron-hungry carcinogen.

The creation of a cancer is a step-by-step process, often requiring many years. The first step is the initial alteration of DNA by a carcinogen, a process known as initiation. A lag of 10, 20 or more years often follows in humans before the deadly fruits of the initial change become evident. During the intervening time, chemicals called promoters enhance the transformation of the altered cell into a cancer. The promoting agent can be the carcinogen itself or another chemical that is not itself capable of causing cancer.

In 1941, the phenomenon of promotion was discovered when a scientist painted benzo(a)pyrene, a carcinogen found in cigarette smoke and the smoke from wood and charcoal fires, on the skin of mice. When one application was placed on the mice, few skin tumors developed. If, after the carcinogen was applied, the skin patch was repeatedly painted with croton oil, a fatty oil from the Indian croton plant and a substance known to be toxic but not carcinogenic, many tumors developed. Oils and fats, components of the American diet that have been linked to an increased risk of colon cancer, are thought to act as cancer promoters and not as initiating carcinogens. Alcohol may also be a promoter of throat cancer, although there is some evidence that it is an initiating carcinogen as well. Cigarette smoke has substances that both induce and promote cancer.

Contact with a promoter over a long period of time eventually causes the affected cell to begin to multiply rapidly, forming a clump made up of nothing but copies of the original cell. This clump grows unchecked, somehow overriding the controls that normally keep cell division from getting out of hand.

A quarter of all Americans now alive will get cancer. Nearly 70 percent of those will die from it. Many of those cancers, perhaps up to 90 percent, will be caused by environmental agents, a growing proportion of which are substances people have added to the air, water, food and land. Many of these substances are known to cause cancer in test animals. A great many others have not been adequately evaluated and hundreds of other compounds are added to the environment each year. While scientists work feverishly to unravel the secrets of cancer and find cures for this terrible killer, people invent new and dangerous chemicals, market billions of pounds of inadequately tested compounds, dump millions of pounds of carcinogens in landfills and water supplies, spew millions more into the air and add millions more to food—forever stacking the deck in favor of this deadly disease.

TESTING: SEPARATING GOOD
CHEMICALS FROM BAD

Knowing how chemical compounds cause adverse effects in the body is only one part of the job of modern environmental toxicology. Another involves determining which chemicals will cause those effects, in what amounts they are dangerous and under what circumstances. How do scientists find out, for example, that one chemical can damage the kidneys or liver while another causes mutations that may lead to birth defects and a third alters the genetic code of cells, resulting, 20 or 30 years later, in cancer?

To determine whether chemicals are harmful, they must be tested on living organisms. For moral, legal and practical reasons, very little of this testing is done on human beings, though it is the effects of chemicals on people that the tests must ascertain. Instead, the testing is done on a variety of animals, ranging from one-celled bacteria to monkeys.

Complementing the animal studies is a science known as epidemiology. Epidemiologists chart the frequency of diseases among the human population and its various subgroups and attempt to find links between the diseases and factors in the environment. As you will see later, epidemiological research is an important way of verifying and expanding the results of tests done with animals.

Toxicologists use whole animals for their studies to simulate the human response to environmental agents. Tests using whole animal models fall roughly into two categories: acute and subacute tests. The most common acute test is simply a measure of how lethal a substance is. Known as the median lethal dose or LD_{50} test, it involves giving two or more species of animals large amounts of a substance to find the dose that will kill half of the test population over a given period of time. The lethal dose is usually calculated in terms of the amount of the substance per kilogram of body weight.

Acute tests allow scientists to determine how toxic a particular substance is compared to other agents and also allow scientists to determine how much of the substance to administer in subsequent studies, called subacute tests. In these, animal models are exposed to smaller doses of the agent every day for about three months to measure the effects of the chemical on the animals. Three dose levels are commonly studied and the animals, generally two species of rodent (mice and rats), are carefully followed throughout the trial period. At the end of the test, all surviving animals are killed and dissected to determine how the chemical acted on various organ systems.

If subacute tests show that a chemical is toxic at smaller, repeated doses, the next step might be to conduct a lifetime test in which the effects of the chemical are studied over the entire life span of the animal (2 to 3 years for a mouse or rat; 7 to 12 years for a dog). Again, the animals are carefully monitored throughout the test and dissected at the end. Since it might take a long time for some chemicals (heavy metals, for example) to accumulate to toxic or lethal levels and because carcinogens typically have long latency periods, lifetime tests may be the only way to ultimately determine whether many substances are harmful or safe.

The design of these tests, including the use of control animals, which are not exposed to the chemical and can therefore provide a baseline with which to compare the reactions of the exposed animals, is critical if the results are to be meaningful. But just as important is the choice of an animal model. All animals have certain fundamental characteristics in common, from the chemical code in their genes to the remarkably consistent structure and biochemistry of their cells. But different species of animals also differ from one another, and from people, in many important ways. For this reason, scientists generally cannot make direct comparisons between animals and people.

Sometimes scientists can determine the nature and magnitude of the differences and then use this information to make extrapolations from animal to human. This process involves estimating the human response based on the reaction of animal models. For example, the rate at which over 100 physiological processes—such functions as respiration, heartbeat and the metabolism of toxic chemicals—take place varies very predictably according to body weight. The smaller the animal, the faster the processes occur. Therefore, the responses of one species can usually be accurately extrapolated from the response of other species.

But many metabolic differences are not as easily predicted across species. For example, the dye benzidine is carcinogenic in rats and humans but not in hamsters. Hamsters seem to metabolize benzidine very differently than the other two species, which may account for the difference. This type of metabolic difference is not usually predictable in advance and causes toxicologists numerous problems as they attempt to determine if animal models truly predict the human response.

There is a great variety of interspecies differences. For example, rats and dogs are more efficient than people in excreting chemicals into their digestive tracts along with bile. Humans are less likely than rats to absorb compounds through the skin. Many chemicals pass more easily through the placentas of rats than through those of monkeys or humans, making rats more susceptible to birth defects. Understanding these differences can help scientists extrapolate from animal to human, and it helps scientists to choose animal models that accurately represent the aspects of the human organism they want to study.

For a fairly long list of reasons, the most popular model for toxicological studies, and in fact for nearly all experimental work with animals, is the rat. The rat is a relatively hardy animal that is not too expensive and is very convenient to use. In contrast to mice, rats are large enough to provide sufficient blood for multiple toxicological assessments. In addition, rats that have been bred to have specific characteristics or specific genetic flaws can be procured in populations in which each rat is virtually a genetic carbon copy of every other rat.

But the rat is far from a miniature version of the human organism and as an animal model it has its flaws. For example, since it was first used as a laboratory animal nearly 100 years ago, the albino Norway rat has been molded by selective breeding to be more adapted to life in the lab. As a result, it is not the animal it once was. Formerly a lean and aggressive creature, suspicious of strangers and highly sensitive to sounds and movement around it, the laboratory rat is now a calmer and stouter creature that is more tolerant of newcomers and more indifferent to changes in its environment. There have been important physical changes as well. For example, the lab rat has smaller organs, including a smaller brain, than its evolutionary forebears.

Many scientists have wondered if this much-changed, highly-tampered-with animal is still suited for the kinds of research the toxicologist must perform. The answer seems to be a tentative yes, at least for qualitatively predicting the human response to environmental agents.

A growing debate among researchers concerns not the validity of using whole animals such as the rat for experimentation, but the necessity. The argument is two-sided. On the one hand are both scientists and lay persons who believe that a great deal of work with whole animals is unnecessarily cruel. Studies in which cosmetics are applied to the eyes of rabbits to test for irritation or in which rats are fed large quantities of a chemical with a stomach tube (called gavage) to test for carcinogenicity are examples of kinds of research that are considered potentially painful or distressing to animals.

On the other hand, there are manufacturers of chemicals and

government agencies that must decide if the hundreds of new chemicals introduced each year are safe. They would like to see less reliance on whole animal tests because they are costly and time-consuming. Groups on both sides of the issue have called for more short-term tests that do not involve whole animals.

One area where short-term tests have proved quite useful is in the determination of whether chemicals have the potential to cause cancer. Traditionally, scientists have tested for carcinogenicity by administering a chemical to groups of male and female rats or mice over a period of two or more years and then comparing the incidence of tumors in the experimental animals with that in a group of control animals. It is a costly and lengthy process.

In the last 20 years, it has become apparent that many carcinogens appear to act by causing mutations. Compounds that can cause mutations, it is generally believed, are also capable of causing cancer. Therefore, carcinogens can often be detected indirectly by tests that measure for mutagenicity. A number of these tests are quick, simple and inexpensive.

The simplest way to begin to evaluate the likelihood that a substance may be a carcinogen involves comparing its chemical structure with those of other substances that are known to cause cancer or mutations. This technique has created a theoretical component of toxicology known as the study of structure-activity relationships. This field holds great promise for markedly streamlining the process of evaluating new chemicals.

Potential mutagens and carcinogens can also be easily screened by determining their ability to cause mutations in bacteria. The most widely applied bacterial assay is called the Ames test. Developed by Bruce N. Ames and his colleagues at the University of California at Berkeley, the test begins with a strain of *Salmonella* bacteria. This particular strain must have the amino acid histidine in its food source to survive. A billion or so of the bacteria are mixed with a chemical to be tested and poured on a Petri dish coated with a growth medium that contains too little histidine to sustain life.

If the chemical under study is a mutagen, it can be expected that it will mutate some of the bacteria on the dish to forms that can make their own histidine and that, no longer requiring the amino acid in the growth medium, will grow and divide. Each mutated bacterium will multiply into a colony visible to the naked eye in the space of a day or two. The greater the number of colonies that turn up, the more strongly mutagenic the compound is.

Unfortunately, the basic Ames test will not detect mutagens, called promutagens, that must be activated through some conversion process in the body. To make the test more realistic, an extract from mammalian liver cells is added to the culture. The enzymes from the extract are thought to act like enzymes in the animal's liver and chemically activate potential mutagens into their destructive form.

In addition to the Ames test, several other short-term assays using bacteria have been developed that can indicate the presence of specific types of DNA damage. Other genetic changes can be detected with short-term tests that employ yeast, fruit flies and cultures of mammalian cells. These include chromosomal aberrations, such as the rearrangement or duplication of entire sections of individual chromosomes, and the presence of extra chromosomes. Some tests can sense the types of chemical reactions that take place only in cancer cells.

No single short-term test can adequately prove whether a substance is or is not a mutagen and, therefore, a likely carcinogen. A positive or negative response in any one test must always be viewed with a healthy degree of skepticism. Many scientists have advocated that any suspected carcinogen undergo a battery of short-term tests. With a well-designed battery, even if one or more tests yield a false positive or a false negative result, the erroneous finding should be obvious when the findings of the battery are taken as a whole.

The results of a set of five or six carefully selected and complementary short-term tests can be an excellent indicator of the potential carcinogenicity of a compound. On the other hand, it can be argued that some compounds may behave differently in a functioning animal than in a bacterium or a tissue culture. Although it is unlikely, a chemical that does not seem to be carcinogenic in the short-term tests may cause cancer in a rat or monkey, so whole-animal tests may still be required before a chemical is pronounced a carcinogen or a noncarcinogen.

No matter how well designed, a test with an animal or a bacterium or a battery of short- and long-term tests can only serve as an approximate model of the human response to the environment. In many ways, human beings are unique, and the validity of such tests, no matter how vital they may be, will always be a matter for controversy among the scientific community and the general public. While many of the questions about these tests center on their ability to predict how people will respond to environmental agents, there are other, equally profound concerns.

For example, if laboratory tests do successfully mimic the human organism, which humans are they simulating? Do they represent the average person, and if so, just what is an average person? Is it a healthy person or a sick one? Does it represent a white or a black; an American Indian or one of Asian descent? Is it a young person or an elderly one? Is it one with a genetic disorder? Is it one who lives in a city or one who lives on a farm? One who dwells in affluence or one who suffers in poverty? One who eats an inadequate diet or a health food advocate? Is it asking too much for animal assays to represent a population as diverse as the human race, or are we all alike enough under the skin for scientists to make meaningful generalizations from animal tests and other types of research?

Another question, one that is often posed by those who must regulate society's use of chemicals, is how well these tests define human risk from environmental agents. Is it possible, for example, to feed large amounts of a food additive to rats and then determine from their response the level at which that chemical will be dangerous to humans? How can the reactions of a six-ounce laboratory rat be compared to the response of a 120-pound human being? Can one accurately extrapolate the risk encountered by a person exposed to a small amount of a poison from a study that involves feeding hamsters, rats or mice amounts thousands of times greater (per pound of body weight) than the average human dose?

There are no easy answers to these questions. Predictive toxicology deals not with certain answers, but with estimates and probabilities. Those who study environmental pollutants must make certain fundamental assumptions about the validity of their work and then attempt to verify those assumptions beyond a reasonable doubt. For instance, it is currently assumed that there is no safe level of exposure to carcinogens. Therefore, the argument goes, it is valid to test for carcinogenicity by exposing animals to extremely high doses of chemicals because if large doses of the chemical cause cancer, smaller, more realistic doses will also cause cancer although in a smaller proportion of the population. The scientist uses very high doses because results can be obtained using a small number of animals. Detecting the cancer-causing ability of a chemical with very small doses could take a great many animals, possibly making the experiment too expensive to conduct. Using the principles of extrapolation, researchers can then mathematically estimate the cancer risk to humans.

While this argument is accepted by the EPA and the FDA, it has also been found to have important limitations. For example, it fails to consider that small amounts of chemicals may behave differently in the body than large doses. In addition, the body's metabolic systems, which can effectively deal with tiny amounts of a chemical, may be overwhelmed by much larger amounts. Factors like these can be important in determining whether a chemical will be a human carcinogen.

LOOKING AT HUMANS

One way to expand on and verify the results of short- and long-term animal assays is to study humans directly. This is the province of the science of epidemiology. The epidemiologist spends his time looking for the causes of human disease. Unlike the medical detective, who may rely heavily on work with animals or on the study of tissue samples from diseased individuals, epidemiologists study the frequency of diseases among various groups of people and then look for circumstances in the lives of those people—their diet, their habits, their jobs—that might provide clues to the causes of the disease.

Epidemiological research generally proceeds in a step-by-step fashion, taking the epidemiologist closer to establishing a cause-and-effect relationship between the environment and the disease with each step. In the first step, the epidemiologist notices that a particular group of people has an unusually large incidence of a certain disease. Next, the epidemiologist looks for factors in the environment that may be causing the disease. He may discover, for example, that one environmental factor seems to be associated with the affected group but not with another, healthier group. Or he may see that a single factor is present in several unrelated groups of people who all suffer a similar incidence of the disease. In other cases, he may see that characteristics of the disease are similar to those of another illness that is known to be related to environmental factors. With this information the epidemiologist can predict the chances of other people becoming ill from exposure to the same environmental agents. These predictions are vitally important to government regulators who must make decisions about the safety of chemical agents and about reasonable limits for human exposure to them.

A major problem with epidemiological studies is that research with people is much harder to control than a laboratory experiment with animals. Where animals can be fed controlled diets and exposed to precisely measured amounts of environmental agents, people lead less ordered lives. Their intake of nutrients is likely to vary widely from day to day and they are exposed to many toxic and carcinogenic chemicals on a regular basis. Three types of studies are conducted in an effort to compensate for some of these problems.

The first is called a case-control study. Case-control studies deal with individuals rather than large groups. Information on diet and exposure to an environmental agent is collected from people who have a specific disease, for example a type of cancer. This information is compared to data gathered from a group of control individuals who do not have the disease. Differences in exposure between the groups not due to chance may indicate a causal relationship between the agent and the disease.

A similar but more sophisticated technique is called the cohort study. A group of subjects is selected, none of whom have the disease in question at the start of the study. The subjects are followed for a long period of time while information on diet or exposure to a chemical or frequency of a certain behavior (like smoking) is collected at regular intervals. At the end of the study, the occurrence of disease among the subjects is correlated with the data on diet or exposure to determine whether the two factors are linked. Cohort studies are performed less frequently than case-control studies because they consume more time and money.

A final, rarely performed study is the experimental or intervention study. In this type of work, volunteers are placed randomly into experimental and control groups and then exposed (experimental) or not exposed (control) to the environmental agent under study. This is the closest scientists can get to a laboratory experiment with people. Intervention studies are most often used to test the effectiveness of new drugs.

Epidemiological studies that evaluate the effects of nutrition on the body's reaction to environmental agents require accurate information on food intake. This is determined in a number of ways. The individual in a household responsible for food preparation may be asked to supply researchers with information about food purchases or menus over a period of time. Often, the individuals in the study are asked to recall what they ate during the past several days or are asked to maintain a diary of their intake over a specified period of time. Sometimes subjects may be asked to fill out a questionnaire describing how frequently they consume certain types of foods.

Each method of obtaining information about diet has its drawbacks. Household records assume that all members of a family consume the same amounts and types of food. Subjects who fill out a diary are likely to change their eating habits, often to make the diary-keeping easier. Methods that ask subjects to record information on just a few days' worth of eating habits may produce unrepresentative information.

HOW RISKY IS IT?

Industry, government and society are making increasingly greater demands on the toxicologist and the epidemiologist. Within recent history hundreds of children have been born deformed because their mothers used thalidomide or developed rare forms of cervical and testicular cancer because of a drug called diethylstilbestrol (DES), which their mothers took to prevent miscarriages. Military personnel in Vietnam and people who live near utility power lines have been exposed to Agent Orange, a defoliant that contains a contaminant known as dioxin, one of the most toxic substances known. Millions of women have in their breast milk the legacy of decades of liberal use of chlorinated pesticides. Across the country, landfills have become secret dumping places for hazardous chemicals and a bewildering variety of toxic and carcinogenic compounds have turned up in drinking water, food and the air we breathe. How dangerous are the compounds that pollute our world? What risks do we face from the thousands of new compounds that are created year after year? Faced with an increasingly risky world, people want answers.

Using the methods described in this chapter, scientists are attempting to find those answers. But scientists must work in the real world. There is just so much time to study each potentially hazardous compound and just so much money to devote to such studies. Limited by time, budgets and the ballooning chemical arsenal, scientists must attempt to learn as much as they can from the tests they have at their disposal in the most efficient manner and weigh the strengths and weaknesses of each type of test.

To understand how environmental agents affect human beings, it is best to study humans directly. For one thing, there is no need to extrapolate from one species to another. For another, there is usually (though not always) less need to extrapolate from grossly high levels to more realistic exposure levels.

The major disadvantage with epidemiological work is that people, for obvious reasons, cannot be manipulated like laboratory animals. This means that scientists must estimate how much of a particular chemical people are exposed to or rely on subjects to report on their exposure. In studies of cancer, the long latency periods between exposure to a carcinogen and the development of the disease make it extremely difficult to say with confidence that the exposure and the cancer are causally related.

Some of the problems inherent in epidemiological studies can be eliminated with animal tests, the most widely accepted means of determining the relative toxicity or cancer-causing ability of chemical compounds. Long-term studies of animals, usually over the lifetime of the animal, are the best way to model the human response to environmental agents. But whole animal studies have important drawbacks. To obtain a toxic or carcinogenic reaction in the test animals, scientists often use large doses, sometimes several thousand times the typical human dose.

This means that the response to realistic levels of the chemical under study must be statistically estimated. Unless suspected carcinogens are tested on more than one species, their cancer-causing ability may be missed, since some chemicals may cause cancer in one species and not in another. But the most important limitation of long-term animal studies is their price tag. A single such experiment can range in cost from a few thousand dollars to well over a million dollars.

Short-term tests have a few important advantages over long-term assays. They can be conducted in a very short time, often just a day or two, and they are far less expensive. They are also easier to interpret and equally if not more sensitive to the toxic or carcinogenic potential of chemicals. Bacterial tests such as the Ames assay are useful for quickly determining whether a compound causes mutations and is therefore a likely carcinogen. In fact, there is a high degree of correlation between findings of mutagenicity in the Ames test and determinations of carcinogenicity in animal tests. Unfortunately, bacteria, yeast cells and fruit flies are poor models of higher animals like human beings. They cannot take into consideration the effects of such processes as absorption of chemicals through the digestive tract and excretion through the urinary system. In addition, it is difficult to determine the magnitude of the risk chemicals pose to humans with short-term assays, so their greatest value is in screening compounds to determine which ones should be further studied with long-term tests and epidemiological studies.

The science of studying the human response to environmental contaminants has progressed remarkably in the last few decades. Better epidemiological methods, more accurate long-term bioassays and more effective short-term tests for mutagenicity have been developed. But there is still a lot to be learned. Government regulators and industries will continue to demand faster, more accurate and less expensive ways to evaluate chemicals. Citizens will continue to demand that they be protected from chemical hazards. The sciences of toxicology and epidemiology will likely advance to meet the demands placed on them. If new compounds continue to be churned out at the current rate, they will certainly have to.

CHAPTER 5

A Chemical Feast:
Our Not-So-Wholesome Food

In the biblical story of Job, it is pointed out that those who sow wickedness reap the same. From pesticides to PCBs, heavy metals to hydrocarbon carcinogens, people have been seeding the environment with chemical wickedness for many generations. And it has followed all too frequently that what we put into the earth turns up later in our food.

Over the years, there have been many horror stories about the toxic bounty on our dinner plates, from reports of mercury in tuna to revelations about DDT in breast milk. Not all poisons in food come from human sources, though. As the first section of this chapter emphasizes, some potent carcinogens are produced naturally.

As food is something we cannot live without, most people have reacted to news about harmful substances in their food either by avoiding foods that might be contaminated or simply by accepting the risk as a fact of life. There is another alternative, though, and that is understanding that the nutrients in food can reduce the likelihood of becoming ill from exposure to these chemical toxins and carcinogens. On a positive note, there is even evidence that a few manmade compounds, such as the additives BHT and BHA, may prevent the cancers caused by environmental agents, as you will see below.

AFLATOXIN: POISON IN THE PANTRY

Though you probably never realized it, you may have one of the most potent cancer-causing agents ever discovered in your home.

If you want to know where to find it, don't bother browsing through the insect killers, paints or automotive products in the garage. And you won't find it under the kitchen sink. If you want to know where to look, try the pantry. That's right, the pantry.

Inside most jars of peanut butter sold in America is a minute quantity of a natural poison called aflatoxin. Also found on corn and grains, aflatoxin is a waste product of a fungus known as *Aspergillus flavus*. Given sufficient moisture, *Aspergillus*, which is closely related to the bread mold that makes penicillin, will proliferate on certain grains and nuts. As it grows, it excretes aflatoxin, which is then soaked up by its host.

Aflatoxin acts primarily on liver cells, although it has also been linked with cancers of the kidney, colon, lungs and lacrimal (tear) glands in animal tests. It was discovered in 1960 after the sudden deaths of thousands of young turkeys in England. Autopsies showed the cause of death to be massive liver damage. Through a bit of medical detective work, the damage was traced to the toxin excreted by the *Aspergillus* fungus, which had heavily infested a shipment of Brazilian groundnuts fed to the turkeys.

Later, aflatoxin was found to cause liver cancer in trout, ducks and ferrets. Epidemiological studies have demonstrated that, with little doubt, the substance acts in a similar fashion on people. In certain areas of Africa, Asia, India and the Philippines, there are pockets of people who suffer the highest incidence of liver cancer in the world. They also eat diets that contain generous portions of nuts contaminated with the *Aspergillus* fungus.

Once the dangers of aflatoxin were recognized, steps were taken in the United States and other developed countries to reduce consumer exposure to this substance (in most Third-World nations few precautions, if any, are taken). By protecting growing crops from damage, which can predispose the grain or nut to infection, storing the harvested crops in cool, dry conditions, and carefully inspecting them before they are processed, the quantity of aflatoxin in American foodstuffs is being kept under control.

But under control does not mean eliminated. Even with stringent regulations and the best quality control, certain foods, especially peanuts, continue to be contaminated. In fact, the Food and Drug Administration (FDA) standard set in 1973 permits aflatoxin in food up to a level of 20 parts per billion. If you were to eat about 15 one-pound jars of peanut butter contaminated with

20 parts per billion aflatoxin in one year, or about three peanut butter sandwiches a week, your chances of getting liver cancer would be estimated as about one in 83,000.

To reduce your risk from aflatoxin, you can, of course, stop eating peanut butter, peanuts and grains. But there may be a more acceptable alternative. Adequate nutrition seems to be important in fighting off this poison. Deficiencies of at least two nutrients may put you at higher risk from aflatoxin.

In 1966, a curious similarity between the characteristics of liver cancers in certain African populations and aflatoxin-induced cirrhosis of the liver in male baboons that had been fed a diet deficient in pyridoxine, a B vitamin, was noted by H. Foy and coworkers and published in the British journal *Nature*. Foy hypothesized that the Africans also had a pyridoxine deficiency that increased their susceptibility to the aflatoxin in the groundnuts they frequently ate. Evidence to support this hypothesis came in 1968 when Paul Newberne and his associates at the Massachusetts Institute of Technology found that rats raised on a diet deficient in certain B vitamins, including pyridoxine, and exposed to aflatoxin were more likely to develop liver cancer than similarly exposed rats fed adequate amounts of the B vitamins.

In separate research, Newberne and his colleagues attempted to determine the effect of vitamin A on the occurrence of aflatoxin-induced cancers. They found that, as with pyridoxine, a deficiency of vitamin A increased the odds of experimental animals' getting cancer—not of the liver, though, but of the colon. Having adequate amounts of vitamin A in the diet is all the more important, the scientists found, because aflatoxin can deplete the body's supply of this nutrient. The results of the work of Newberne and others have a clear message for peanut butter eaters—eat a diet rich in vitamin A and pyridoxine (see Chapter 3). Peanut butter, by the way, is a poor source of both of these nutrients.

Interestingly enough, peanut butter may contain built-in protection against the natural carcinogen it contains. Peanut butter is naturally high in unsaturated oils. In research with animals, fats, particularly unsaturated fats, were found to reduce the amount of aflatoxin absorbed through the digestive tracts of chickens. More research is needed to find out if the oils in peanut butter afford people the same type of protection.

NITRITES AND NITROSAMINES: A RISKY REACTION

Aflatoxin represents a class of poisons that are naturally present in food. Fortunately, natural toxins, especially those from poisonous plants or spoiled food, are usually easy to avoid. But, as if to compensate for nature's lack of toxic pitfalls, people have peppered their food with a host of hazardous materials. Many are deliberately added to food to preserve it, stabilize its color, flavor it, tint it, make it sweeter and reduce bacterial contamination.

Sodium nitrite is a compound commonly used to color and preserve cured meats. The use of this nitrite began over 100 years ago when it was noticed that salt, once the most common preservative, turned patches of meat pink. It turned out that the color was due not to the salt, but to sodium nitrite, a contaminant of the salt. Meat vendors soon began to add sodium nitrite to cured meats to give them a uniform pink color, but what established nitrite's popularity was the discovery that it had a remarkable ability to prevent the growth of the bacteria that cause botulism.

All this would have remained an interesting bit of history had it not been discovered in the late 1960s that various nitrites can combine with another class of organic chemicals, amines, to form nitrosamines, some of which are extremely powerful cancer-causing agents. This chemical reaction takes place to a limited extent when meats are processed, as they sit on the grocer's shelves and, especially, as you cook them. But the reaction can be speeded up by placing the ingredients in an acidic solution, like the juices in the human stomach.

It does not take a chemist to mix nitrites and amines in the right proportions. Any pizza maker can do it. A pepperoni pizza contains enough nitrites in the sausage and an ample supply of amines in the dough to make a respectable batch of nitrosamines. You can, of course, increase the odds by throwing in more amines in the form of beer or wine and more nitrites packaged as ham or smoked anchovies, but a pepperoni pizza (or a breakfast of bacon, eggs and toast, for that matter) will do the trick.

You don't have to rely on the alchemy of the kitchen or the biochemistry of your stomach to be exposed to nitrosamines, though.

Nitrosamines have been found in beer and wine, certain cosmetics and even baby bottle nipples. In March of 1982, the United States Food and Drug Administration reported that it had detected minute amounts of these carcinogens in rubber nipples, though it said the risk to babies was very small, and it was not considering a ban or recall.

Once ingested or manufactured in the biological flask of the stomach, nitrosamines are absorbed into the bloodstream and transported to sites in the body where they can induce cancer. In studies with animals, various nitrosamines have been found to cause cancers of the liver, kidney, lung, stomach, esophagus, bladder, nose, intestine and tongue. Few other carcinogens attack as many organs and systems as nitrosamines.

There is no direct evidence yet that nitrosamines cause human cancers, though the indirect evidence is strong. For instance, esophageal cancer among Bantu men in Africa is believed to be caused by the practice among tribesmen of curdling milk with fruit juice contaminated with nitrosamines. Zambians, who drink alcohol with one to three parts per million nitrosamines (enough to cause cancer in animals) also have a high rate of cancer of the esophagus.

Evidence also exists which suggests that nitrosamine-induced cancer can be prevented with nutrition. A deficiency of zinc, for instance, seems to increase the risk of esophageal cancer, and inadequate intake of B vitamins may elevate the risk of all types of nitrosamine-induced cancer. But the best way to combat these carcinogens is to prevent them from entering the body at all.

Extensive research has shown conclusively that vitamin C can prevent the formation of nitrosamines in the stomach. This phenomenon was discovered quite by accident in 1972 when S. S. Mirvish and his colleagues at the University of Nebraska were trying to confirm an earlier report that the antibiotic oxytetracycline, an amine, could combine with nitrites to form nitrosamines. The first time they tried the experiment the results were disappointing. When the researchers noted that the drug had been formulated with a large amount of vitamin C, they decided to try again with pure antibiotic. This time they produced nitrosamines as expected.

Surprised by the ability of vitamin C to block the amine-nitrite reaction, the researchers decided to study the phenomenon in more detail. In experiment after experiment, this remarkable property of vitamin C was confirmed and reconfirmed. From the body of evidence collected to date, it appears that vitamin C competes with amines for any available nitrite. By combining chemically with the nitrites, vitamin C prevents their transformation to carcinogens.

Although the amount of vitamin C required to deactivate a certain amount of nitrites in the human stomach is not known, in animals the ratio is generally two parts ascorbic acid to one part nitrite. Since nitrites are present in meats in very small amounts (the federal limit on the amount of nitrites in food is 200 parts per million), a glass of orange juice contains more than enough vitamin C to counteract the nitrites in an average meal.

More research is needed to confirm the value of vitamin C as a cancer preventer in humans, but a study conducted by A. J. Varghese and his associates at the University of Toronto in 1978 offered a hint of proof. In that study, a human subject agreed to take a vitamin C supplement for a period of several weeks. The researchers measured the quantity of carcinogenic nitrosamines in his feces for a week before and two weeks after the supplementation began.

As predicted, the nitrosamine level in the feces dropped 70 percent after the subject began the vitamin C treatment and returned to normal when the treatment was stopped. Studies like this have convinced some scientists that foods treated with nitrites should be fortified with vitamin C to prevent the formation of nitrosamines. In addition, numerous drugs that contain amines should be formulated with vitamin C to prevent them from combining with nitrites in the digestive tract.

Interestingly, preliminary studies conducted in the late 1970s indicate that vitamin E may be more effective than ascorbic acid in preventing the conversion of nitrites and amines to nitrosamines. Vitamin E can reduce the amount of nitrosamines in fried bacon when the vitamin is added to fresh pork bellies and can prevent the formation of nitrosamines in cigarette tar if it is added to cigarettes.

The data on vitamin E is in need of a great deal of verification. However, the evidence clearly indicates that vitamin C can block the chemical reaction that yields the carcinogenic nitrosamines.

We can strongly recommend that any meal which includes pre-pared meats, such as cured ham, pepperoni and sausage, or smoked fish be accompanied by vitamin C. The best way to do this is to eat an orange or drink a glass of orange juice *before* the meal so the vitamin C is waiting in the stomach for the nitrites.

DES: A TROUBLED SAGA

In 1971, a disturbing finding was reported in the pages of the *New England Journal of Medicine*. A rare form of cervical and vaginal cancer, known as clear cell adenocarcinoma, was being seen in a small number of young women, though this rare form of cancer had previously been reported almost exclusively in women over 50.

The cancer that struck these women and the testicular cancer that afflicts a small number of men as well had little if anything to do with what these individuals had done during their lives. Instead, it was caused by a substance their mothers had taken while pregnant. These were the DES daughters and sons, victims of diethylstilbestrol, a drug used until the 1970s to prevent miscarriages, even though its effectiveness was never proved. Tragically, the drug, a synthetic female sex hormone, crossed the placentas of the pregnant women who took it and affected the genetic material of their developing children. For about one in 1,000 of those fetuses, the result was cancer.

The use of synthetic estrogens like DES is also known to increase the risk of uterine cancer in women who take them for the treatment of menopausal symptoms and certain types of cancer. In fact, though no longer prescribed for pregnant women, DES is still used for these purposes. All of this would be an interesting, and compelling, medical sidelight except for one very troubling fact. Whenever you eat beef, you are consuming DES.

Cattle growers have known for quite some time that DES increases the weight gain of a cow. For years, they have administered the drug to cattle by placing DES pellets into the ears of the animals while they undergo their final fattening-up period. In 1980, the practice was interrupted by a federal ban on the use of DES in cattle, but the ban was lifted a year later and the FDA now permits the drug to be used as long as no more than one person in one million can be expected to get cancer by eating beef contaminated with DES.

One puzzling aspect of the cervical, vaginal and testicular cancers induced in the DES daughters and sons is the relatively small number of exposed offspring who ultimately developed cancer. Though it is estimated that between 500,000 and 2 million American women used DES between 1950 and 1970, less than one percent of their children have developed cancer as a result of the exposure. By comparison, nine percent of American women get breast cancer. Nutrition may partly explain this anomaly.

As far back as 1949, researchers began to study the effect of dietary fat on the rate of mammary cancer in mice exposed to DES, which was known to be a carcinogen long before its effects on offspring were discovered. The researchers kept rats on high and low fat regimens and fed them DES. Substantially more tumors developed in rats fed the high-fat diet, and the tumors developed more rapidly than the cancers affecting the rats in the low-fat condition.

Unfortunately, no one has followed up on this intriguing finding, so it is difficult to say how significant diet is in human susceptibility to DES. However, as we will note in Chapter 9, diets high in fat have been shown to be almost unquestionably linked to the development of certain types of cancers, including breast and uterine cancers. The relative levels of certain types of natural estrogens also play a role in the development of these cancers. Therefore, it would not be at all surprising if DES, a synthetic estrogen, and dietary fat interacted to promote cancers.

Those who are exposed to DES either as a prescription drug or as a food contaminant might benefit from lowering their overall consumption of fat. Since beef is a high-fat food, it would be best to limit beef consumption to extra-lean cuts and very lean hamburger—that with less than 15 percent fat.

BHA AND BHT: PRESERVING MORE THAN FRESHNESS

The case of the common food additives BHA and BHT departs somewhat from the other stories in this chapter. Instead of unwanted contaminants or health-threatening additives, these are compounds that may have beneficial effects that go far beyond what the food processors who use them might imagine.

Both BHA (butylated hydroxyanisole) and BHT (butylated hydroxytoluene) are members of a class of food additives known as synthetic antioxidants. They are mixed with processed foods to keep fats and oils from turning rancid and to prevent the changes in color, texture and flavor that occur when food is exposed to air. Synthetic antioxidants are added to a wide variety of foods, including bread and many other grain and cereal products. They are even included in the cardboard of the boxes that many breakfast cereals are packaged in. Americans consume about two milligrams of synthetic antioxidants every day, most of it as BHA and BHT.

In 1972, L. W. Wattenberg from the University of Minnesota discovered that these two additives do more than maintain the freshness of foods. In a study with rodents, Wattenberg found that BHA and BHT could prevent the induction of mammary and forestomach cancers caused by two common carcinogens. Since that study, several researchers have extended the list of carcinogens that these additives will counteract. Other work has suggested that they may prevent the noncarcinogenic toxic effects of certain other chemical compounds and even prevent viral infections.

BHA and BHT are two of several antioxidants that are able to alter the activity of a group of enzymes in the liver known as the mixed function oxidase system. These enzymes are thought to convert harmful or potentially harmful chemicals to less harmful substances. BHA and BHT may help the liver enzymes deactivate cancer-causing chemicals.

BHA and BHT may also act directly on certain compounds. For instance, in a 1975 experiment Wattenberg and a colleague noted that benzo(a)pyrene, a known carcinogen, was kept from binding with the DNA of mice fed BHT. The researchers assumed that since the carcinogen was unable to alter the DNA, it would be unable to initiate a cancer. In other studies, both additives have been found to speed the excretion of carcinogenic chemicals.

Because the work on BHT and BHA has been carried out on animals and not humans, it is difficult to say for sure that these chemicals act the same way in the human body, though there is no reason to believe they do not. According to Wattenberg, the average daily intake of BHT and BHA by adults (about two milligrams) is enough to protect against two milligrams of a carcinogen like benzo(a)pyrene. By coincidence, two milligrams is just about the average amount of benzo(a)pyrene people receive from vegetables, open fires, charcoal grills, cigarette smoke and other sources each day. If this is true, then BHA and BHT may have already made their mark as cancer preventers. In fact, some scientists believe the wide use of these antioxidants may explain the drop in the rate of stomach cancer in the United States in recent decades.

PCBs: A PERSISTENT THREAT

In this century, there have been many tales of chemical substances introduced by proud chemical companies and heralded as wonder compounds. They fill dozens of niches formerly occupied by more expensive products and, the icing on the cake, they do their jobs even better than their predecessors. For years, they quietly make our lives easier and their manufacturers richer.

Then it happens. First in the medical journals, then in the popular press, word begins to appear that all is not right. The wonder chemicals cause cancer, promote heart disease or induce birth defects. There are denials by the manufacturers, skepticism by government regulators and a growing body of damning evidence. Finally, after months or years of controversy, the compounds are quietly taken off the market or banned. Lingering long after the last drop or ounce leaves the factory is always the same question: How, with a regulatory mechanism designed to protect consumers from just this type of hazard, could a time bomb like this slip through?

Perhaps one of the most notorious time bombs of recent years has been a collection of organic chemicals known as polychlorinated biphenyls, or PCBs. Introduced in the mid-1930s, PCBs were soon serving a variety of useful purposes. As solvents, sealants, hydraulic fluids, adhesives, lubricants, heat transfer fluids, plasticizers, carriers for pesticides and dielectric oils in transformers and capacitors, they easily fit the criteria for wonder compounds. In 1970, about 80 million pounds of PCBs were manufactured in the United States and an estimated 50 million pounds were lost to the environment through spills, leaks and deliberate dumping from manufacturing plants.

Like many chlorinated substances (see *Chlorinated Pesticides* below), PCBs are slow to break down in the environment. They accumulate in the waterways where they are dumped and turn up in increasing amounts in fish, birds, poultry, milk and human beings. About ten percent of United States women may have potentially toxic levels of PCBs in their breast milk.

The pervasiveness of PCBs is troubling in and of itself, but it becomes a chilling fact when added to the knowledge that these compounds are highly toxic and can cause cancer in laboratory animals. Because of this, PCBs are no longer manufactured, and the federal government is funding the development of safe methods to destroy the millions of pounds of PCBs still in use in transformers and other large electrical equipment. Though the PCBs are sealed inside electrical equipment, they can still be a hazard. A 1981 fire in a transformer vault of a Binghamton, New York, office building, for example, contaminated several firemen, numerous onlookers and a clean-up crew with PCBs and their toxic by-products.

Even if all of the PCBs still in use were safely disposed of, these compounds would remain a major health problem. Millions of pounds of PCBs are in the environment and will remain there for generations. They will continue for years to turn up in our food and will build up, day by day, in our body fat. There is evidence, though, that we do not have to be totally helpless victims of PCB contamination. Nutrition, in particular vitamins A and B_{12}, may help protect the body against these carcinogens.

When a large dose of PCBs is given to a rat, the animal's store of vitamin A declines, sometimes dramatically. In one experiment, rats fed one type of PCB lost 50 percent of their reserves of vitamin A. In individuals with adequate nutrition, this may not pose a major health threat, but it can be quite serious for those with a marginal vitamin A deficiency. Attempts to determine how PCBs diminish the body's stores of vitamin A have not yet yielded a definitive answer. Experimental results have suggested that the chlorinated compounds keep the body from manufacturing a protein that normally binds with vitamin A in the blood. PCBs may also promote the destruction of vitamin A in the liver.

A serious consideration for scientists is the potential consequence of this induced vitamin A deficiency. Vitamin A is necessary for the normal growth of a type of tissue known as epithelium. It is known that less than optimal levels of vitamin A in this tissue might predispose the body to chemically induced cancer (see Chapter 9). Could PCBs, by lowering the amount of vitamin A in the body, reduce the body's resistance to the carcinogenic action of PCBs and other environmental agents? Unfortunately, the research that could answer that question has yet to be performed.

One sign of PCB poisoning is a blemishing of the skin. Coincidentally, the same skin disorders are characteristic of a deficiency of various of the B vitamins. In 1977, two researchers decided to determine if this coincidence could shed any light on the effect of PCBs on the human body. After feeding PCBs to laboratory animals for a period of time, the scientists measured the quantity of vitamin B_{12} stored in their bodies. As they had expected, the researchers found that vitamin B_{12} levels dropped significantly after the PCB exposure. Further work revealed that PCBs act in a similar fashion on thiamine, another B vitamin. Because the amounts of PCBs fed to the rats were several times higher than what people normally encounter, it is not known how seriously PCBs might affect a human's requirement for B vitamins.

Despite the inconclusiveness of the evidence with regard to PCBs and vitamins A and B, it does suggest that one way to reduce one's odds of getting sick from exposure to PCBs is to eat a diet rich in both vitamin A and the B vitamins. In fact, since PCBs seem to induce deficiencies of both vitamins in animals, it may be wise to consume somewhat more than the recommended daily intake of both vitamin A and vitamin B_{12}, although more research is needed to confirm this.

CHLORINATED PESTICIDES: SILENT KILLERS

Like PCBs, chlorinated insecticides are extremely persistent in the environment. The most famous and notorious member of this class of chemical poisons is known by the tongue-twisting scientific name of dichloro-diphenyl-trichloroethane. Most people know it as DDT. Introduced in the 1940s, DDT rapidly became the pesticide of choice. Tests in Switzerland, where it was first marketed, revealed that it could kill all manner of insect pests while not being highly toxic to people or other higher animal life.

After a successful tour of duty in World War II, where it fought off malaria-infested mosquitoes and held down the cholera and typhus that had plagued soldiers in previous wars, it was rapidly adopted by the agricultural industry in the United States and soon spread all over the world. Millions of pounds of this cheap and easy-to-use pesticide were applied to fields every year. Through runoff and seepage into the soil, it found its way to waterways and into the food chain. Like PCBs, DDT is now a part of the tissues of most living things.

Since they are stored in the fatty portions of animal bodies, both DDT and PCBs are now found in appreciable quantities in dairy products and in human milk. Several studies in the United States and Canada have found high levels of both types of compounds in breast milk. The levels of DDT have often exceeded the acceptable daily intake set by the World Health Organization. In fact, the quantities in some women are high enough to make the milk unacceptable for sale had it come from a cow. (The story is no better for PCBs, and in fact surveys have shown that about ten percent of American women have amounts of PCBs in their milk high enough theoretically to cause toxic reactions in infants.)

Though DDT is not highly poisonous, its toxicity is still of concern to public health officials because this chemical does tend to build up to high concentrations in human beings. Also of great concern is the fact that DDT is carcinogenic in mice and is suspected of causing cancer in people as well. It is estimated that at a concentration of ten parts per billion—a reasonable estimate of the average body burden of Americans—DDT could be expected to account for about 63 excess cases of cancer every year. When the federal government finally moved in the early 1970s to ban the aerial spraying of DDT except where necessary to protect public health, other chlorinated pesticides gained in popularity. With names like chlordane, dieldrin, mirex, kepone, Heptachlor and lindane, these proved just as persistent and, for a few of them, several times more toxic than DDT. Many of these, too, have been banned.

In recent years, chlorinated pesticides have faded from popularity in favor of the somewhat less effective though more biodegradable organophosphates, such as malathion, parathion and naled. But, just as with PCBs, a decline in the quantities of chlorinated pesticides entering the environment does not eliminate the danger these compounds pose to people. Lingering in the soil, water and our food is a menacing residue of DDT that will remain for years to come.

In 1971, two scientists at Utah State University took two seemingly unrelated facts and developed a hypothesis that provided intriguing evidence that vitamin C may help protect the body against the toxic effects of DDT and other chlorinated pesticides. D. J. Wagstaff and J. C. Street noted that pesticides, like other foreign chemicals, are detoxified or made less poisonous by the actions of liver enzymes. They also observed that a deficiency of vitamin C can reduce the effectiveness of these enzymes. So they exposed guinea pigs raised on an ascorbic-acid-free diet to several chlorine-containing pesticides. They found that as the levels of vitamin C in the animals' bodies dropped, the ability of the animals to deal with pesticides diminished in step.

Recognizing that a complete absence of vitamin C in the diet is an extreme rarity, Wagstaff and Street evaluated the potency of the detoxification mechanism at various levels of dietary ascorbic acid. They found that the ability to stimulate the liver enzymes that deactivate chlorinated hydrocarbons increased as the amount of vitamin C ingested rose. Interestingly, quantities of the vitamin sufficient to prevent scurvy did little to spur the activity of the enzymes. Enzyme stimulation occurred only after these levels were exceeded several times over. Amounts considerably in excess of the recommended dietary allowance seemed able to sustain the enzymes' activities at still higher levels.

Other research has suggested that a deficiency of vitamin C slows the removal of chlorinated pesticides from the body. As yet, there has been no thorough evaluation of the significance of this line of research to humans, although there is reason to believe that vitamin C levels may be related to the detoxification and excretion of these compounds in people as well. In light of the widespread exposure of people to pesticides, more studies are needed.

Whereas vitamin C may aid in the removal of chlorinated pesticides from the body, the poisons themselves seem to do the same thing to vitamin A. After reports in the 1950s and 1960s of vitamin A deficiencies in cattle in areas where chlorinated pesticides and herbicides were used heavily, researchers began to study the effects of pesticides like DDT on the vitamin A requirements of animals. Although there was some disagreement about the results, early studies seemed to indicate that exposure to chlorinated pesticides not only brought on outward signs of a vitamin A deficiency in cattle and other animals, but also caused measurable decreases in the liver vitamin A stores. Further work demonstrated that although chlorinated insecticides may decrease the body's supply of vitamin A, there was probably little to be concerned about in terms of human health. Examination of the livers of Canadians during autopsies in 1977 found no relationship between vitamin A level and the amount of pesticide in the organs.

Several studies since the Canadian investigation have offered conflicting evidence on the effect of pesticides on vitamin A stores. Although the effects on humans, as several researchers suggest, may be minor, there is evidence that even these minor effects can be alleviated. Proteins, in particular proteins that contain the sulfur-based amino acid methionine, protect the body's supply of vitamin A from pesticides. Studies with animals suggest that a higher-than-normal protein intake may enhance this effect, but the significance of this work to humans is not yet known.

Much work has been directed at finding ways to remove pesticides from the body. Some exotic techniques have been tried with animals, but these are not recommended for humans. Starvation diets, for example, free pesticides from fat deposits, but the sudden jump in the amount of poison in the blood can cause a severe toxic reaction. This has been demonstrated in test animals placed on a starvation diet after consuming sizable quantities of insecticides. These animals developed insecticide-induced nerve tremors as their bodies began using pesticide-laden fat deposits for food.

Unfortunately, there has been little work to date on the ability of nutritional factors to speed the removal of pesticides from the body. In studies with cattle, supplements of vitamins A, D and E did virtually nothing to remove chlorinated pest killers from the animals. Vitamin E purged the pesticides from certain tissues, but the overall level in the body remained unchanged.

While vitamins may not be able to cleanse the body of pesticides, it is apparent from the research described in this section that one vitamin, C, may be able to help the body detoxify these poisonous and potentially carcinogenic substances. The research found that vitamin C seems to act by stimulating the activity of the liver enzymes that break down the pesticides. Since these same enzymes also deactivate many other chemical poisons, the benefits of eating a diet high in vitamin C will go far beyond protecting the body from pesticides. How much vitamin C one should consume to achieve optimal protection from pesticides is not known. Animal research seems to indicate that it is higher than the RDA for the vitamin, which is only designed to fend off scurvy. Whether megadoses will prove any more useful in stimulating liver enzymes than moderately large doses is, again, not known.

For women who may be worried about potentially unsafe levels of pesticides and other hazardous substances in their breast milk, the only sure way to find out if breast milk is safe is to have it tested. At the moment, this may be difficult, as state and regional public health laboratories are not geared up to do routine human milk testing. But your local public health agency should be able to tell you how you can have your milk checked out.

MERCURY: A TAINTED FISH STORY

"Shun mercury as poison" if you suffer from scurvy. That was the proclamation of nineteenth-century London physician George Budd, who believed that a deficiency of vitamin C markedly enhanced the toxicity of mercury. It was an intriguing suggestion that would wait more than 100 years to be put to the test. It appears to have been excellent prophecy.

In 1951, M. Vauthey showed that a certain dose of mercury cyanide killed all of the rats it was administered to in one hour. If the rats were given extremely high doses of vitamin C (equivalent to 35 grams for a human, or about 580 times the recommended dietary allowance for a human adult), 40 percent of the animals survived. Four years later, two researchers showed that vitamin C administered before or along with a dose of mercury-based diuretic reduced the incidence of toxic side effects, such as cardiac arrest.

Most of us are aware of mercury's unusual properties, which have made it an object of special fascination for scientists and a boon to manufacturers, and also of its extreme toxicity. The only metal that is liquid at room temperatures, mercury has found a multitude of niches in modern industry. It is the silver liquid in thermometers, a component of many drugs, the gas in mercury vapor street lights, the electrical conductor in many electric switches and a component of dental fillings. But one common use has spread the insidious poison through the land and sea.

Before they were banned in 1976, mercury pesticides were sprayed in huge amounts on American crops. These pest killers were made from organic methyl mercury, which is many times more poisonous than the inorganic, metallic mercury. Approximately 800,000 pounds were sprayed onto fields in 1971 alone. Several accidental poisonings by the pesticides or contaminated seeds alerted officials to the extreme danger these mercury compounds posed to people. Unfortunately, the damage had already been done. Heavy pesticide use and indiscriminate dumping of mercury compounds resulted in widespread environmental pollution by methyl mercury. As a result, mercury has found its way into the food chain. Absorbed by ocean-bottom–dwelling bacteria, which are eaten by algae, which are eaten by small fish, and so on, mercury can eventually accumulate in very large amounts in such fish as tuna and swordfish. Although there is debate about how much mercury these fish would pick up from natural sources if there were no pollution, there is little doubt that mercury in the diet can pose a health hazard.

That vitamin C can affect this hazard was suggested by a 1974 study by Susan Blackstone and her colleagues in Great Britain. She found that elevated levels of vitamin C in the diet diminished the amount of mercury in certain tissues and seemed to reduce its toxicity. Unfortunately, large amounts of vitamin C in the diet also seemed to increase the intestinal absorption of mercury, suggesting that it may actually enhance mercury poisoning. As a result, Blackstone has strongly recommended that anyone who may be exposed to significant amounts of mercury avoid taking megadoses of vitamin C. Dr. Orville Levander of the United States Department of Agriculture recently echoed Blackstone's suggestion.

Selenium, a mineral required in very small amounts (about 50 to 200 micrograms per day), has been shown in several animal studies to counteract the effects of ingested mercury. Selenium is a gray, nonmetallic element known to electrical engineers as the substance that forms the heart of photoelectric cells. Initial findings in the 1960s that this mineral might offer some protection against the harmful effects of mercury spurred a flurry of interest. At least 50 original research projects have been mounted to study this interaction. In 1967, J. Parizek and I. Ostadalova, noting that selenium can protect the body against cadmium—an element that behaves similarly to mercury in the body—fed high levels of both mercury and selenium to rats and found that animals fed selenium suffered less kidney and intestinal damage than rats who received no selenium.

Parizek's results were later confirmed and expanded by other studies. In all cases, however, the amounts of mercury used greatly exceeded what most people consume. In addition, the protective doses of selenium were also many times greater than the normal daily human intake. In some cases, the selenium doses would in themselves have been toxic to humans. Results like these make it difficult to predict how well supplements of selenium may guard people against mercury at normal or even higher-than-normal doses.

One study, however, may bode well for people who like to eat tuna, swordfish and other large fish that have been known to contain methyl mercury. Although it is not yet known why, selenium often seems to accumulate along with mercury in animals. Noting this, a team of researchers fed Japanese quail diets consisting either of tuna that contained both mercury and selenium or of corn and soya to which mercury was added. While 54 percent of the quail that ate the mercury-contaminated corn-soya diet perished, only 7 percent on the tuna diet died. The results indicated that the selenium in fish may offer built-in protection against mercury.

The protective effect of selenium is a promising development in the long saga of mercury toxicity. The story for vitamin C is, on the other hand, complicated by the effects of large doses of the vitamin, which may actually increase the toxic effects of mercury on the body. In fact, as noted above, researchers have strongly cautioned against those who are routinely exposed to mercury taking megadoses of vitamin C. As for selenium, most of us get enough of this mineral in our normal diets. However, those who suspect that their diets are low in selenium, those who eat a great deal of fish or those who are frequently exposed to mercury might want to think about taking a daily 50-microgram supplement.

CONCLUSION: SAVING GRACES

It is discouraging to realize that food, the stuff that sustains life, can also pose a threat to our health. Aflatoxin in peanut butter, mercury in fish, nitrites in cured meat, DES in beef and chlorinated compounds in nearly everything make one wonder just how safe it is to eat in our modern world. For while we can avoid certain foods we know may be contaminated, we can never completely reduce the exposure to toxins and carcinogens that we receive through food.

Fortunately, some foods contain built-in antidotes to the chemical hazards they bear. The oils in peanut butter, for example, may reduce the effectiveness of the carcinogenic aflatoxin that peanut butter contains. Fish contains selenium, a mineral that may offer some protection from mercury. Processed foods frequently contain additives known as BHT and BHA, which may protect the digestive tract from chemical carcinogens in food, and in fact are thought to be largely responsible for the declining rate of stomach cancer in this country.

Thus, an important way to protect oneself from many of the toxins and carcinogens in food is with good nutrition. Deficiencies of certain vitamins and minerals can place one at a heightened risk to a variety of environmental hazards. For example, deficiencies of vitamin A or the B vitamin pyridoxine can increase one's susceptibility to aflatoxin. Too little zinc or B vitamins in the diet can elevate the risk posed by nitrosamines. A deficiency of vitamin C may leave one at a greater susceptibility to the ubiquitous poison DDT.

Some hazards in food are capable of causing vitamin deficiencies. Both DDT and PCBs, for example, cause vitamin A deficiencies in test animals. PCBs can also cause deficiencies of thiamine and vitamin B_{12}. In only a few cases do nutrients present in unusually large quantities increase one's risk from poisons or carcinogens in food. A diet high in fat can increase the odds of getting cancer from DES. Very large doses of vitamin C may increase the toxicity of mercury.

Only one well-researched and well-understood case of a nutrient offering nearly complete protection from a poison in food is yet known. It has been shown that vitamin C, when present in the stomach with a meal containing nitrites and amines, can prevent the formation of the highly carcinogenic nitrosamines. In fact, any meal that includes cured meats or smoked fish should be accompanied by a glass of orange juice or an orange. Ideally, the orange or juice should be consumed just before the meal so the vitamin C is in the stomach waiting for the nitrites when they arrive.

The science of determining just what one should eat to protect onself against the environmental contaminants one consumes is, as much of this chapter suggests, still in its infancy. In fact, the federal RDAs, which are the standards for determining the quantity of nutrients we require each day to stay healthy, do not yet take into consideration the beneficial effects many nutrients have in counteracting pollutants in food. The research conclusions described in this chapter cannot be taken as definitive dietary guidelines; many of the results were obtained with animal research and have yet to be adequately confirmed in human trials. However, since deficiencies of nutrients generally seem to enhance the effects of pollutants in food, it is clearly important to eat a diet that contains at least the recommended levels of all nutrients.

CHAPTER 6

No Escape: Pollutants in
Our Air, Water and Land

—In Contra Costa County, a community near San Francisco
dotted with over 40 oil refineries and chemical plants, residents awake to another day of foul-smelling smog that
often burns the nose and throat.

—In communities along the Niagara River in upstate New
York, over 300,000 people drink water that may be contaminated with a variety of potent organic carcinogens that
enter the river, their drinking water source, from dozens
of chemical plants in the area.

—In a large housing development outside of Washington,
D.C., a group of children make mudpies in a backyard
that borders a major interstate highway. The dirt in this
yard is contaminated with lead from the exhaust of the
thousands of cars and trucks that pass by each day.

—In a refurbished farmhouse in Amherst, Massachusetts, a
woodstove takes the chill off a winter evening and fills the
air with carbon monoxide, nitrogen dioxide, benzo(a)pyrene
and many other toxic and cancer-causing chemicals.

For most of us, whether we know it or not, pollution is virtually a constant companion. When we breathe, we are likely to inhale at least trace amounts of toxic gases or particulate matter,
whether on the job, in our homes or in the great outdoors. When
we drink a glass of water, we may very well be sipping a solution

that contains lead, cadmium, copper, asbestos or a variety of organic chemicals. Even the dirt in our gardens and backyards may be laden with heavy metals.

An unfortunate aspect of this type of pollution is that we are often not even aware of it. Improperly disposed-of chemicals can seep out of municipal landfills and into our wells. Gas ranges can silently fill a kitchen with dangerous levels of carbon monoxide. Unless we have our water or air tested, we may never be the wiser.

Though we may not notice the environmental contaminants around us, they can be a hazard to our health. According to a survey by the National Center for Health Statistics, about four percent of all preschool children and an unknown number of older children and adults suffer from subclinical lead poisoning. Hundreds of thousands of cases of environmental illness (from allergic responses to cancer) that occur every year are believed to be due to the presence in our drinking water of organic chemicals such as chloroform and trichloroethane or to the use of wood-stoves, fireplaces and kerosene heaters that contribute carcinogens and other harmful agents to the air in our homes.

Because pollutants are so prevalent in our world, it is imperative that we find ways to protect ourselves from them. Many claims have been made in recent years that proper nutrition may help reduce our chances of succumbing to diseases, including those caused by environmental agents. This chapter will examine some of the pollutants that threaten our health and some nutrients that may reduce, or enhance, our susceptibility to them. We will evaluate a variety of nutrient and pollutant interactions to see which have held up to scientific scrutiny.

LEAD: THE SUBTLE CRIPPLER

It is a blue-gray metal known for its malleability. Fashioned into products as diverse as fishing weights and shields for radiologists, it is one of the most widely used metals in industry. It is an ingredient in automobile batteries, a lining for storage tanks and pipes, a component of paints, glazes, enamels, glass and solder, and an antiknock agent in gasoline.

Its many applications have made lead at once a boon to modern society and a scourge to public health. Lead is a highly poisonous substance. In relatively small doses, it can cause flulike symptoms. Ingesting greater amounts may cause intense pain in the abdomen and joints and the destruction of red cells in the blood, which leads to anemia. In severe cases, lead will attack brain cells, causing symptoms ranging from disorientation and irritability to mental retardation.

Sometimes the signs of lead poisoning are subtle. In 1979, Dr. Herbert Needleman and his colleagues at the Harvard Medical School measured lead levels in the baby teeth of over 3,000 schoolchildren in two towns in Massachusetts and then checked their performance on tests that measure intelligence, verbal and speech skills and attention span. Even slightly elevated lead levels were associated with lower test scores. In addition, the more lead in the teeth, the more likely it was that teachers, who were not aware of the students' lead levels, reported that the children were easily distracted, hyperactive, daydreamers, unable to follow simple directions, disorganized and so on. The learning problems continued as the children got older, a follow-up study a few years later concluded.

Children are at very high risk to lead. They absorb lead through their digestive tracts much faster than adults, and the blood-brain barrier, which prevents harmful substances from entering the brain, is much more porous in the very young than in adults, making them more sensitive to lead-induced brain damage. In addition, children are more likely than adults to eat lead-contaminated soil, swallow leaded paint chips or encounter lead in many other ways.

The Pervasive Poison

Unfortunately, there are far too many ways for children and adults to come into contact with lead. After it is mined, lead gets into the environment right away as rain washes it from mine tailings into the ground and waterways. Later, lead enters the air from smelter and manufacturing plant smoke and in the exhaust from cars and other vehicles burning leaded fuel. There is also lead in the smoke from burning cigarettes. About 600,000 tons of lead spew forth into the atmosphere each year, about 90 percent of that from automobile tailpipes.

Though most new cars use unleaded fuel, there are still many older models on the road that use leaded gas. In fact, about half of the gasoline now made still contains small amounts of lead. Until recently, refiners were able to put an average of half a gram of lead per gallon in their gasoline. Since this was averaged across all of their gas production, half of which was unleaded, the limit actually allowed about one gram of lead in the leaded grades. New regulations proposed by the EPA in 1982 should lower the amount of lead in each gallon of leaded gas and, therefore, reduce the amount of lead that enters the atmosphere from cars. In fact, the EPA predicts that the new regulations will reduce lead emissions from cars by as much as 31 percent. But that still means that hundreds of tons of lead will belch forth each year.

A very heavy element, lead eventually settles out of the air and becomes a permanent part of the soil. Lead in the soil may be a big contributor to our body burden of this toxic metal, particularly in cities and other heavily trafficked areas. Various studies have shown that a teaspoon of dirt in inner-city playgrounds in Los Angeles or New York City can have up to 3,000 micrograms of lead, ten times more lead than an average child can safely ingest in a day.

Air pollution is not the only source of lead in the soil. The extensive use over the years of pesticides made with lead compounds has left many farms and much former farmland heavily contaminated. House paint was also once an important source of lead in the soil. Before 1940, some paints contained as much as 50 percent lead. In the years after the mid-1950s, other compounds were found to replace lead as a drying agent and pigment and the concentration of lead in paint declined. The 1971 Lead-Based Paint Poisoning Prevention Act set the maximum allowable level of lead in paint at 1 percent. In 1973, the limit was dropped to 0.5 percent and then in 1977 it was dropped again to 0.06 percent.

Although modern paints contain less lead than older paints, they are still a hazard, and an unnecessary one at that, since other substances can be used instead of lead. And, though you can no longer buy high-lead paints, old, heavily leaded paint still coats the walls in many buildings, especially in poorer urban areas. When this paint flakes and falls off walls or when walls of old buildings are torn down, the lead can become part of the dust and soil.

Peeling paint is still a major cause of lead poisoning in young children. Naturally curious and fond of placing nearly anything in their mouths, babies and toddlers are understandably attracted to paint chips. If the paint they eat is very old, they may consume in a few tastes enough lead to cause serious brain damage. Even if they do not ingest paint, the dust and dirt kids normally get on their hands can also contain lead, especially in houses in cities or near busy roads.

Lead is also commonly found in drinking water. Various surveys of drinking water supplies across the United States have determined that the average amount of lead in water is about 13 micrograms (millionths of a gram) per liter. One obvious source of this lead is pollution. Automobile exhaust can settle onto reservoirs, especially those near highways. Steel mills, iron foundries, zinc mines, battery makers and other industries all contribute lead to the environment, as do municipal landfills. The refuse from our daily lives—tin cans, old batteries, paint cans, construction and demolition debris—can all leach lead into nearby reservoirs and aquifers.

But only a portion of the lead that ultimately comes out of the tap is there when the water begins its journey to the faucet. As the water passes through mains and household plumbing, more lead is picked up. In the Northeast, Northwest and other areas of the country that have soft water that is slightly acidic and high in dissolved oxygen, a significant amount of lead may leach from waterpipes. In a 1975 EPA study of water in Boston and Seattle, two cities that have corrosive water, between 65 and 76 percent of the water samples were found to exceed the federal drinking water standard of 50 micrograms of lead per liter. The highest lead levels were found in the early morning after water had been sitting in the household pipes for several hours, suggesting that it is a good idea to let the water run for a few minutes before filling the teakettle or the coffeemaker in the morning.

People who live in new homes or in houses that have seen a few harsh winters may be at a higher-than-average risk of lead exposure. The pipes in most homes are held together with a solder that contains at least some lead (many are 50 percent lead), which can leach into the water. The greatest amount of lead seeps out when the solder is new. Although the amount of lead leached from solder drops as a house gets older, in cold climates this trend is often counteracted by burst pipes, which must be mended with fresh solder.

An adult who drinks two liters of water daily ingests about 20 to 30 micrograms of lead each day along with his or her drinking water. Children consume anywhere between 5 and 15 micrograms. However, the amounts contributed by drinking water are dwarfed by the quantities of lead normally found in the average American diet. It is estimated that adult men consume about 300 micrograms of lead in their food each day. Women and young children daily ingest about 100 to 150 micrograms. But, while adults absorb only 5 to 10 percent of the lead they eat through their digestive tract, children take 40 to 50 percent of the ingested lead into their bodies.

Soil and airborne lead can coat fresh fruits and vegetables. Animals raised for meat pick up lead from their feed and water supplies. Lead is also inadvertently added to food during processing and cooking, especially if the food is prepared in lead-contaminated water. Canned foods are a very important source of lead. Most cans used to hold processed foods consist of a sheet of tin-coated steel rolled into a tube. The end pieces of the can are crimped on mechanically, but the seam of the steel tube is sealed with a bead of lead solder. About two-thirds of the lead in canned food comes from this lead seal.

In the early 1970s, the Food and Drug Administration started a program to reduce the amount of lead in canned foods, concentrating first on foods canned for children. A particular concern was evaporated milk, then widely used to make infant formulas. The side seams as well as the top and bottom seams and a small vent hole of the milk cans were sealed with lead, which resulted in canned milk having a higher percentage of lead than most canned foods.

In 1973, the evaporated milk industry began to reduce the amount of lead in their product, complying with an FDA limit of 0.5 part per million (ppm). In fact, by 1982 the lead content of canned milk had dropped far below the FDA limit, going from 0.52 ppm to 0.08 ppm, an 85-percent reduction. Similar reductions have been achieved with canned infant formula (from 0.1 ppm to 0.02 ppm), glass-packed solid infant foods (from 0.15 ppm to 0.03 ppm) and infant juices, which were once canned and are now largely bottled (from 0.1 ppm to 0.015 ppm). By using more two-piece cans with crimped-on lids and switching to electrically welded seals (see *Protecting Your Family from Lead*, below), canners have also begun to reduce the lead content of canned adult foods, though the reductions have been more modest.

By reducing lead in canned foods, cutting the lead content of paint and pushing refiners to make more unleaded gasoline, the federal government has succeeded in reducing the exposure of the average American to this toxic metal. In 1982, the National Center for Health Statistics reported that the levels of lead in the blood of all Americans had dropped by nearly 40 percent compared with the previous four years. That is an impressive achievement, but it is only the beginning of a long and difficult battle.

Protecting Your Family from Lead

There are many ways parents can reduce their children's exposure to lead. Old paint can be scraped off walls and replaced with lead-free paint. Parents can be careful to select canned foods in two-piece cans (identifiable by their rounded bottoms and lack of a side seam) or cans with nonlead seals (these usually have a black or blue line running down the seam) and also try to serve more fresh and frozen products. Parents can also quit smoking and encourage their children not to take up the habit. When plumbing is installed or fixed, low-lead solders can be used and care taken to do the job neatly. Drinking water and the soil in yards and playgrounds can be tested for lead; and parents can urge their government representatives to introduce and vote for legislation to reduce the risk of lead poisoning by improving programs to detect and treat lead poisoning in children.

There is still another way to combat lead poisoning: proper nutrition. Lead interacts with many nutrients. Some decrease its absorption into the body and some increase it. Others affect the rate of excretion of lead or its toxicity. Understanding how nutrition affects the susceptibility of the human body to lead may ultimately provide a powerful weapon against lead poisoning.

The influence of nutrition on lead poisoning was recognized as far back as the early 1900s. At that time, milk was commonly given to industrial workers who came into contact with lead. How milk came to be thought of as a prophylactic agent is not known, but it was probably believed that as a food rich in nutrients it would improve the generally poor diet of workers. A healthy body, it was believed, would be better able to defend itself against the chemical assault of the workplace.

The value of milk in the fight against lead poisoning has been studied and debated for many years. That numerous studies have yielded confusing and often contradictory results is not surprising. Milk is a complex food made up of many nutrients, including calcium, phosphorus, magnesium, copper, iron, protein, fats, niacin, and vitamins C, D and E. All of these nutrients have been found to affect the toxicity of lead, some offering protection, others enhancing lead's negative consequences.

For example, calcium and lactose are two of the principal ingredients of milk. Calcium markedly reduces the quantity of lead the body can absorb through the digestive tract, thus reducing the amount that can lodge in and damage kidneys and brain cells. Lactose, on the other hand, seems to aid the body's uptake of this poisonous metal. Interactions like these place in question the value of milk in reducing lead poisoning.

That calcium and phosphorus can block the passage of lead from the digestive tract to the bloodstream had been hinted at in the 1930s, though the first studies to offer convincing evidence of this phenomenon were not carried out until years later. Two researchers, Kathryn Mahaffey and Robert Goyer, in 1970 noticed that rats fed a low-calcium diet retained much more lead in their tissues and displayed more pronounced symptoms of lead poisoning than animals with adequate nutrition.

The effects of phosphorus depletion were even more pronounced. Rats fed 70 percent of the required intake of phosphorus suffered effects from lead similar to those suffered by rats fed only 30 percent of their requirement for calcium. When calcium and phosphorus were given to the animals in excess of dietary needs, they seemed to offer extra protection against lead poisoning, especially if given simultaneously and in large amounts. For human beings, though, the most significant aspect of this research is not the benefit of excess minerals in the diet, but the bane of poor nutrition. Rats raised on a low-calcium diet and exposed to lead in drinking water experienced symptoms similar to those suffered by rats fed a normal diet and exposed to nearly 20 times as much lead.

Research with animals also suggests that children who do not eat enough calcium and phosphorus may develop a taste for lead. Rats weaned on a diet low in calcium voluntarily drank solutions of a lead compound, while other rats given adequate calcium found the mixture unpalatable. Similarly, monkeys only marginally deficient in calcium (having about 75 percent of their normal intake) will readily drink a lead solution. If fed sufficient calcium, the same monkeys will develop an aversion to the contaminated water.

This craving for lead may be explained by the fact that lead can take the place of calcium in the body, albeit with unfortunate results. If adequate amounts of calcium are not present in food, the body may make do with lead or other heavy metals. When the body's stores of calcium are low, the production of a protein that binds with this mineral and transports it into the body is stepped up. If there is little calcium to bind with, it will mistakenly latch on to a molecule of lead. However, when both calcium and lead are present in the digestive tract, the protein seems to seek out the calcium and leave the lead behind.

Studies of the average nutrition of children around the country have shown that youngsters most likely to be exposed to lead are also those who are most certain to have deficiencies of calcium and phosphorus. Low-income families, particularly urban blacks and other minorities, are more likely than other families to eat inadequate diets. Children from these families are also likely to encounter old paint chips, play in lead-contaminated soil and breathe lead-tainted air.

Copper, magnesium and iron, like calcium and phosphorus, seem to diminish the absorption of lead when eaten in adequate amounts. On the other hand, deficiencies of any of these nutrients markedly enhance the passage of lead into the body and magnify the effects it has on various tissues. For example, in work with animals, it has been shown that levels of lead in the blood are inversely proportional to the amount of copper in the diet. In addition, lead can reduce the concentration of copper in the bloodstream, increasing the body's need for this mineral. Lead also increases the body's need for iron. Lead seems to slow down the production of hemoglobin and the formation of normal red blood cells. It may do this by interfering with the body's ability to use iron.

To make the hemoglobin molecule, the body must go through a series of steps, creating chemical intermediaries or building blocks along the way. Lead can stop the manufacture of hemoglobin at some of these steps, but the administration of niacin can help prevent lead from throwing a monkey wrench into the body's chemical factory. Rats first given amounts of lead large enough to drastically reduce the production of hemoglobin and then given large quantities of niacin quickly recovered and produced the blood protein at a normal rate. Two other B vitamins, B_6 and B_{12}, also protect the hemoglobin assembly line from lead. In addition, cobalt, which is a part of the B_{12} molecule, can help alleviate lead poisoning.

A deficiency of vitamin E can also lower the amount of hemoglobin in the blood when the body is challenged by lead. While lead in the absence of iron or B vitamins shuts down the production of this protein, insufficient vitamin E combined with lead results in the destruction of red blood cells, the carriers of hemoglobin. Red blood cells are normally pliable. This is important because the capillaries in the spleen, the tiniest pipes in the body's plumbing system, are smaller in circumference than the red cells that pass through them. When these cells reach the spleen, their pliability allows them to squeeze through the tiny passageways unharmed.

In animals deprived of vitamin E, though, the red cells become stiff. Coupling an E deficiency with a toxic dose of lead often results in cellular havoc. The cells turn brown and brittle. The blood undergoes a marked decrease in hematocrit, the portion of blood made up of red cells. Anemia sets in and the spleen enlarges. The red cells, unable to bend as they reach the spleen's narrow passages, are trapped. Eventually, the pressure of the continuing blood flow enlarges the spleen and begins to break up the brittle red cells. Treatment with vitamin E has been effective in preventing this condition in rodents.

The combination of lead and a vitamin deficiency may also be responsible for the deterioration of the blood vessels in the brains of rats exposed to lead. This condition, which usually leads to cerebral hemorrhage in test animals, is the first tentative indication that supplementation with vitamin E may help prevent brain damage in children exposed to lead. This hypothesis is especially interesting in light of the frequency of vitamin E deficiencies among the poor.

There is evidence that vitamin C may be able to prevent the damage lead does to the blood and central nervous system. In the late 1930s and early 1940s, two studies were conducted that involved the administration of small to moderate doses of vitamin C to industrial workers who exhibited symptoms of lead poisoning. It was found that the vitamin supplements improved the health of workers. In particular, the supplements reduced the damage done to red blood cells. A study of house painters who used lead paint showed that vitamin C apparently reduces the entry of lead into the body through the digestive tract.

Since then, work with animals has supported the conclusions of these earlier human studies. One of the most promising research projects was conducted in 1979 by a team led by Dr. Robert Goyer of the National Institute of Environmental Health Studies. In work with rats, they found that vitamin C could combine with lead and remove it from the central nervous system. If this ability of vitamin C is confirmed, the vitamin may prove to be a highly effective treatment for children who are at risk to brain damage from ingested lead. It appears that vitamin C will be most effective if administered along with calcium EDTA, a food preservative that can also remove lead from the body.

While dietary minerals, niacin and vitamins C, E, B_6 and B_{12} may protect against lead intoxication, vitamin D, fats and lactose seem to enhance it. Work with laboratory animals has determined that vitamin D enhances the intestinal absorption of lead and increases the amount of lead that is deposited in bones. However, this effect does not occur if the diet includes adequate quantities of calcium, since vitamin D selectively promotes the absorption of calcium when both calcium and lead are present in the digestive tract.

However, too much vitamin D can enhance the absorption of lead even if one's diet contains adequate calcium. Children can develop an excess of vitamin D during the summer when they play for long periods of time in sunlight, which stimulates the formation of vitamin D in the skin, and when they are drinking more milk fortified with vitamin D. The combination may result in a higher-than-normal uptake of lead. In fact, it has been shown that people who live in the Northern Hemisphere tend to have higher blood levels of lead in the summer. Fats also seem to markedly affect the uptake and retention of lead by the body. A study in the mid-1970s, supporting research done 40 years earlier, found that increasing the level of corn oil in the diet of rats substantially elevated the amount of lead stored in the soft tissues. Another study obtained the greatest increase in lead retention with buttermilk, suggesting that saturated fats are the most likely to increase the uptake of lead. A deficiency of protein also speeds the absorption of lead. In several studies completed over the last 40 years, animals fed a protein-poor diet and exposed to lead exhibited retarded growth and excess lead in the soft tissues. A combination of low protein and high fat was particularly detrimental.

Lactose, the sugar found in milk, can also markedly affect the amount of lead absorbed by the body. Lactose makes up from four to seven percent of the milk of mammals and is an important nutrient for nursing babies. It has been known for several years that this sugar helps the body absorb many essential minerals, such as calcium, iron and zinc. Only recently did two researchers at the University of Wisconsin in Madison discover that this effect also applies to lead. They fed rats a normal diet including various quantities of lactose and then exposed them to lead. Increasing amounts of lactose were associated with larger quantities of lead in the blood, liver, kidneys and bones.

Recent and exciting work done by several Soviet researchers determined that apple pectin, which is derived from the peel of apples, considerably reduced the changes in the blood cells of industrial workers exposed to lead, an effect also seen in tests with animals. The researchers were so impressed, they recommended that all workers exposed to lead eat apple pectin daily.

The amount of pectin in an average apple is probably less than the quantity these workers ate every day, but it seems reasonable to assume that even a small amount of pectin could have a beneficial effect. An apple a day, it turns out, may actually keep the doctor away.

As this section has shown, eating apples is just one of many ways one can increase one's resistance to lead and the symptoms of lead toxicity. In particular, dietary minerals seem to be highly effective in reducing the absorption of lead through the digestive tract, thus reducing the quantities that might reach the tissues of the body. Deficiencies of any of these minerals, particularly calcium and phosphorus, can drastically escalate the effects of lead on the body. For this reason, parents should make sure their children get adequate amounts of calcium, phosphorus, copper, magnesium and iron. Children's diets should also include adequate amounts of vitamins C and E, both of which protect the blood cells and blood-forming organs and both of which may help to prevent brain damage caused by exposure to high levels of lead.

CADMIUM: A USEFUL POISON

Like lead, cadmium is pervasive in the environment. Found in the soil, in drinking water and, primarily, in food, it has become an important threat to public health. Also, as with lead, the prevalence of cadmium is partly due to its many uses in industry. Highly resistant to corrosion, cadmium is often used to protect iron, steel and copper and is frequently released to the environment from metal ore smelters and steel plants. It is also used in photocells, as a coating for welding electrodes, as a plasticizer in PVC products, in pigments—especially yellows and oranges—in the making of jewelry, in control rods for nuclear reactors, in the manufacture of semiconductors and fluorescent lamps and in superphosphate fertilizers.

For most Americans, the main source of exposure to cadmium is the diet. Market-basket surveys by the FDA between 1968 and 1974 indicated that the average American consumes between 26 and 61 micrograms of cadmium each day. About two percent of this is actually absorbed through the digestive tract, although as you will see, certain nutrients can have an important effect on how much cadmium we take into our bodies. Drinking water can be another important source of cadmium. Although most United States drinking water supplies do not have excessive amounts of cadmium, and few in fact exceed the United States EPA standard of ten micrograms per liter, cadmium can be added to water as it passes through distribution systems and household plumbing. This is a particular problem in areas that have soft and acidic water supplies and in areas that have galvanized steel pipe, which always contains at least some cadmium.

Cadmium is also found in cigarette smoke (see the smoking section of Chapter 9). One pack of cigarettes can put between two and four micrograms of cadmium into the lungs, where cadmium is most readily absorbed. Airborne cadmium can also be an important hazard in many occupations.

Overall, the average American is exposed to between 40 and 190 micrograms of cadmium each day. The higher end of that scale represents people who smoke, live in industrialized cities and eat a diet with appreciable levels of cadmium. Cadmium is removed from the body very slowly, in fact in one day's time, only one or two micrograms are excreted in the urine. Consequently, cadmium tends to accumulate in the body over the course of a lifetime. Most of us are born with almost no cadmium in our tissues. By the time we are 50, our bodies contain between 15 and 50 milligrams.

Unlike lead, which is stored predominantly in the bones, cadmium accumulates in the liver and, especially, the kidneys. When the concentration in the kidneys rises above about 200 micrograms per gram of tissue, kidney damage can result. In experiments with rats, rabbits and humans, cadmium has been found to cause lesions in the kidney. It also causes high blood pressure in animals and has been associated with hypertension in people. While the exact mechanism by which cadmium causes high blood pressure has not yet been determined, it is known that cadmium increases the retention of sodium (which has also been linked to high blood pressure), constricts blood vessels and increases the pumping volume of the heart.

In preliminary work with laboratory animals, cadmium has been found to be both a mutagen and a carcinogen. These animal tests have been supported by epidemiological studies that have found associations between the amount of cadmium in drinking water or food in various areas of the country and the occurrence of several types of cancer. It is believed that cadmium may act by inhibiting the intestinal absorption of selenium, a mineral that is believed to have anticancer properties. Though the initial findings are compelling, the National Academy of Sciences, in its 1982 report on *Diet, Nutrition and Cancer,* concluded that the evidence does not yet permit any firm conclusions about the ability of cadmium in the diet to cause cancer in humans.

In several experiments with animals, supplements of zinc have been found to reduce the toxicity of cadmium. In particular, damage to the testes of male rats, which can occur when these test animals are exposed to large amounts of cadmium, was eliminated with zinc supplements, and other types of tissue damage were prevented as well. It is believed that excess zinc may trigger the production of a protein that normally binds with zinc in the bloodstream. Since cadmium binds with this protein even more strongly than zinc, the protein may take cadmium out of circulation and keep it from reaching its target tissues. Supplements of copper have also been found to lower cadmium toxicity.

Some recent research into the toxic effects of cadmium has been spurred by the occurrence in Japan of an affliction known as Itai-Itai disease, which causes bone demineralization and kidney damage in women. Itai-Itai has been linked to cadmium, particularly in those whose diets were found to be low in calcium. Research with animals has shown that a calcium deficiency greatly increases the amount of cadmium that will pass through the walls of the digestive tract. In fact, it has been shown that the amount of cadmium absorbed is inversely related to the amount of calcium in the diet. The protein in the lining of the digestive tract that escorts calcium into the bloodstream seems to also have a strong affinity for cadmium. When the diet is deficient in calcium, more of this protein is manufactured to scavenge as much calcium as possible from the contents of the digestive tract. Unfortunately, this will also increase the absorption of cadmium.

Excess calcium reduces the absorption of cadmium and also alleviates one of the metal's more serious effects. Studies have shown that rats given hard water, which has a high level of calcium, seem resistant to the high blood pressure normally caused by large doses of cadmium. Scientists are now wondering if calcium offers the same sort of protection against hypertension in humans.

Just as with inadequate amounts of zinc or calcium, too little iron can also increase the body's susceptibility to cadmium toxicity. An iron deficiency markedly increases the absorption of cadmium through the digestive tract and aggravates cadmium's negative effects. When mice are given fairly small amounts of cadmium in their drinking water and fed a low-iron diet, they experience a great reduction in both body weight and the number of red blood cells as compared to mice fed a diet with either low iron or cadmium. In a study done with human volunteers in 1978, the absorption rate of cadmium was four times higher in people who ate a diet low in iron when compared with those who ate a normal diet. Women, who as a rule have lower stores of iron than men, especially as a result of menstruation, are more likely to have a significantly greater cadmium absorption. In fact, it has been found that menstruating women as a group absorb cadmium three times as readily as men.

Another important nutrient in the battle against cadmium is vitamin C. Primarily because of the work by Margaret Spivey-Fox and her colleagues at the USDA, we now know that vitamin C prevents or reduces many of the effects of cadmium in laboratory animals. For example, it can prevent cadmium from slowing normal growth; it protects red blood cells and also protects the bones and prevents them from becoming cadmium storehouses. In addition, it can prevent the deterioration of the testes, sperm and bone marrow that cadmium can cause.

Supplements of vitamin C equivalent to 780 milligrams in humans (13 times the recommended daily adult human intake) have been highly effective in preventing cadmium poisoning in guinea pigs, which, like people, do not manufacture this vitamin. Excess vitamin C seems to act by preventing cadmium from depleting the body's iron. Tests have shown that when iron and vitamin C are given in excess together, their individual beneficial effects are multiplied.

Because of the pervasiveness of cadmium in our world, and because of its potential to cause kidney damage and, quite possibly, cancer, it is important that ways be found to lower human susceptibility to this hazardous chemical. The research described in this section has shown that nutrition may be a valuable weapon in the fight against cadmium. In particular, vitamin C and the minerals zinc and calcium can prevent or lessen some of the toxic effects of this heavy metal in test animals. Although these findings await verification in human studies, it is clear that a deficiency of any of these nutrients may place you at a heightened susceptibility to this pollutant.

FLUORIDE: A MINOR BLEMISH ON ITS IMAGE

In 1902, a Colorado Springs dentist noticed that a few of his patients had discolored tooth enamel. Interestingly, the same patients had very little tooth decay. It was not until 30 years later that it was found that excess fluoride in drinking water could account for both conditions. A study done in the 1940s examining tooth decay rates in cities with varying amounts of fluoride in their drinking water supplies found that a concentration of one milligram per liter or one part per million fluoride could markedly reduce the incidence of dental caries. People who drank water with this amount of fluoride had 60 to 65 percent fewer cavities than those drinking water low in fluoride.

After several studies confirmed these impressive results, intentional fluoridation of water supplies was endorsed in the late 1950s by the United States Public Health Service, the American Dental Association and the American Medical Association. In the years since the benefits of fluoride were discovered, fluoridation has been credited with a general improvement in American dental health, particularly among the poor, who cannot afford proper dental care. Despite charges made over the years that fluoridation is a communist plot, a violation of freedom of choice and a possible cancer threat, the practice, which still costs less than 50 cents a person per year, continues to be one of the most inexpensive and effective public health programs ever devised.

In some communities, fluoride occurs naturally in levels that are equal to or higher than the one milligram per liter commonly added in fluoridation programs. A survey of 969 water supplies across the country in 1979 found fluoride levels ranging from 0.2 milligram per liter to 4.4 milligrams per liter. In 1970, a survey by the Dental Health Division of the Public Health Service found that nearly one million people in 524 communities consumed water with more than 2 milligrams per liter. The average American probably consumes a milligram or less of fluoride in drinking water each day.

Fluoride also occurs in food, especially fish and tea. In addition, when food is cooked or processed in water that contains fluoride, its fluoride content increases. It has been estimated that eating canned food, for example, can add about half a milligram of fluoride to one's daily intake. All told, the average American probably ingests about 0.5 to 2 milligrams of fluoride each day in food.

In areas where drinking water contains no fluoride, dentists often prescribe fluoride drops or tablets for children and many schools have established programs to administer fluoride tablets or mouth rinses to students under the age of 12 on a regular basis. And, of course, most Americans use a toothpaste that contains fluoride and dentists routinely give their patients' teeth fluoride treatments.

In regions where fluoride levels are normally high, occasional cases of tooth enamel mottling occur in children. Mottling ranges from opaque white flecks on the teeth to brown stains. Mottling has also been seen in infants and youngsters given fluoride drops and, in fact, the concentration of fluoride in these drops was cut in half in 1982 to prevent this problem. While mottling seems to be relatively common, it does not pose any threat to the children's health.

One fact that has struck researchers studying mottling is how different regions of the country with similar levels of fluoride in the drinking water have different incidences of childhood tooth discoloration. Average climate seems to make a difference. Mottling is less common in colder areas, possibly because children in warm regions drink more water. How much bottled water or beverages children drink and how much processed food they consume can also make a difference. It may also be that parents in certain regions do not consider mottling to be objectionable and do not report it to dentists and doctors.

The variation in the incidence of mottling may also be due, in part, to diet. For example, adequate or elevated levels of calcium in the diet can reduce mottling, while a calcium deficiency can increase it. Vitamin C has also been related to tooth mottling. Studies in the 1930s found that children with the most severe mottling were also likely to have a deficiency of vitamin C.

Knowledge of how these and other nutrients affect discoloration of teeth by fluoride may help reduce or eliminate the only significant drawback of a highly successful public health program. The fluoridation of drinking water has meant a drastic improvement in the dental health of millions of children in the United States, particularly those who are members of families who can not afford proper dental care. Until now, the mottling of teeth in a small number of children who consume fluoride in drinking water or as drops, tablets or rinses has been seen as an unfortunate but necessary part of this health program.

Perhaps by ensuring that their children eat diets rich in vitamin C and calcium parents can prevent tooth mottling from occurring in their children. More work with human subjects will be necessary before this can be shown to be an effective preventive measure. In the meantime, though, by providing their children with good sources of these two nutrients, parents may be protecting them not only from tooth discoloration, but also from more serious toxic effects of lead and cadmium (as was shown in the two previous sections).

ORGANIC CHEMICALS: THE GROWING MENACE

They are clear, colorless liquids, which often have sweet or pleasant odors. Despite their innocuous appearance, they are capable of causing cancer and birth defects in animals and, in some cases, humans. They are called volatile organic contaminants, or VOCs, and they are turning up with increasing frequency in water supplies all across the country. The list of compounds that have been detected in both surface water supplies and wells reads like the index of an organic chemistry textbook. Trichloroethylene, tetrachloroethylene, carbon tetrachloride, 1,1,1-trichloroethane, 1,2-dichloroethane, vinyl chloride, methylene chloride, trichlorobenzene,

1,1-dichloroethylene, cis-1,2-dichloroethylene, trans-1,2-dichloroethylene, benzene, chlorobenzene and dichlorobenzene constitute just a small sample from that list.

Since the United States Congress passed the Safe Drinking Water Act in 1974, the EPA has conducted several major surveys of VOCs in United States drinking water supplies. These have shown that, though most public water supplies are free of VOCs, there are numerous cases of ground and surface water contamination. In one survey of 330 water supplies in 46 states, the EPA found detectable levels in 13 of 29 communities with populations over 10,000 and in 37 of 301 municipalities of less than 10,000.

In Maine, 19 of 87 municipal wells tested in a statewide survey had at least one type of volatile organic contaminant. At least a trace of trichloroethylene or tetrachloroethylene turned up in 210 out of 296 wells tested in California's San Gabriel Valley. In Connecticut, 87 percent of wells serving at least 1,000 residents were found to contain VOCs.

In most cases, the levels detected have been low, but isolated cases of very high contamination were recorded. One well had 35 parts per million of trichloroethylene, a very high level. At least 44 communities in Massachusetts, 25 in Pennsylvania, 16 in Connecticut, 12 in New York and at least one municipality in each of 40 other states have had their public water supplies severely contaminated with volatile manmade organic chemicals.

Where do these chemicals come from? There is no simple answer to that question. One thing is certain, though: None are naturally present in the environment; all are synthesized in factories in huge amounts. For example:

—*Trichloroethylene (TCE)*: Over 300 million pounds of this solvent were manufactured in 1978; about 267 million pounds were released to the environment. TCE is used extensively in industry as a degreaser for metals and as a dry-cleaning agent.

—*Tetrachloroethylene (PCE)*: Over 725 million pounds of this widely used compound were made in 1978; perhaps 606 million pounds were eventually lost to the environment. This compound, which will remain in water supplies for years, is used to dry-clean textiles and to make aerosol propellants, is incorporated into certain pesticides (especially fumigants) and is used as a degreaser.

—*Carbon tetrachloride:* About 739 million pounds were made in 1978 and 96 million pounds lost. It is used as a metal degreaser, a solvent, a dry-cleaning agent and an ingredient in fire extinguishers.

—*1,1,1-trichloroethane:* Over 625 billion pounds were made in 1978; about 533 million pounds were released to the environment. Extremely high levels of this compound have been detected in wells in a few states. Although its primary function is metal degreasing, this compound is also used in leather tanning, as a solvent for adhesives and inks and in the making of pharmaceuticals.

—*1,2-Dichloroethane:* About 11 billion pounds of this widely used compound were made in 1977 and nearly 80 million pounds lost. It is used in the manufacture of other organic chemicals, as a gasoline additive and a solvent. Despite its large production, it has not been detected in many wells sampled in EPA surveys.

Volatile organics are released to the environment during manufacture, storage and shipping. Much of the loss, though, probably occurs when they are actually used by various industries and businesses. Tragically, though, a great deal of VOC pollution can be chalked up to improper disposal of these compounds.

Literally millions of pounds of volatile organics, many known or suspected carcinogens, have been carelessly dumped in sanitary landfills that are not designed to hold them. Newspaper reports of dumps loaded with leaky 50-gallon drums of hazardous waste seem to crop up with greater and greater frequency. The case of the Love Canal area of New York is certainly the best known example of poorly handled industrial waste, but it appears that there may be a great many other Love Canals all across the nation.

Large quantities of VOCs—the exact amount will never be known—do not make it to landfills. So-called midnight dumpers, usually small companies hired to transport waste to treatment facilities, have been known to dump their cargoes far short of their goal, occasionally right into lakes or streams that serve as drinking water sources. A lack of adequate treatment plants for organic wastes and the high cost of properly disposing of these chemicals are the reasons often cited for the occurrence of midnight dumping.

The frequency with which these chemicals are found in United States drinking water supplies makes it all the more important to understand how diet can affect the toxicity and carcinogenicity of VOCs. Unfortunately, little work has been done in this area, and data on only a few volatile organic compounds are available. In the next chapter, Chapter 7, we will review research that has examined nutritional interactions with benzene, carbon tetrachloride, vinyl chloride, chloroform, 1,2-dichloroethane and 1,2-dichloropropane. Two other types of organic chemicals, chlorinated pesticides and polychlorinated biphenyls (PCBs), are also widely found in water supplies, food and human beings. These were discussed in Chapter 5.

OZONE, NITROGEN OXIDES, BENZO(A)PYRENE, RADON AND OTHER AIR POLLUTANTS: AN ILL WIND

A popular 1981 movie dealt with early man's first energy source. Called *Quest for Fire,* the film might just as well have been titled *Origin of Air Pollution.* Since people first learned to burn fuel to cook food and heat dwellings, we have been fouling the air with the by-products of combustion. Air pollution became serious business as large towns and cities brought many people, and many pollution sources, into close proximity, and when fossil fuels, such as coal, replaced wood as primary heat sources. Today, air pollution is a major threat to public health, especially in urban areas, where residents are often faced with smog alerts, choking smoke, or acrid fumes.

Though we once thought of air pollution as something we encountered outside our homes, recent studies have shown that the quality of air in our dwelling places may be a greater health risk. Furnaces, stoves, fireplaces, cigarettes and the chemicals we use to clean our homes can all contribute poisons and carcinogens to the air we breathe. Even the materials we use to construct our homes can contaminate our indoor atmosphere. Urea formaldehyde insulation can leach formaldehyde, a suspected carcinogen, ceiling and floor tiles can contribute asbestos fibers and stone and brick can give off radioactive radon gas.

In this section we will look at both varieties of air pollution—

indoor and outdoor. We will also examine some ways nutrition may help protect us from air pollutants and how, in fact, the food we eat may be one of our best weapons against the hazards in the air around us. We will start with outdoor pollution.

Air Pollutants in the Great Outdoors

The histories of certain cities have been marked by catastrophic or near-catastrophic episodes of air pollution. For example, between October 27 and 31, 1948, 43 percent of the 14,000 population of Donora, Pennsylvania, sought medical attention and 17 people died as a temperature inversion over the city trapped sulfur dioxide, smoke and zinc compounds from two mills and a sulfuric acid plant. Between 3,500 and 4,000 people died in London on four days in December 1952 as a pea-soup smog of smoke and sulfur dioxide settled over much of the United Kingdom. A total of 1,700 died in two other pollution episodes in London in 1956 and 1962.

These were highly unusual events, but everyday pollution in major cities also takes its toll in life and health. In metropolitan centers like Los Angeles and New York City, smog is an accepted evil of city life. Pollution alerts punctuate the typical summer day. But foul air is no longer limited to cities. Prevailing winds can transport pollutants hundreds of miles. In addition, transplanted industries, automobile-clogged suburbs and an alarming rise of wood-burning in rural areas have made air pollution an almost inescapable phenomenon. While most people suffer the inconvenience of tainted air with seeming indifference, the aged, the very young and those with respiratory disorders often wage a life-threatening battle with the very air they breathe.

Air pollution is a complex blend of many noxious chemicals. Its sources are many and range from burning leaves to major industries. The most important contributors to atmospheric filth are fossil fuels—oil, coal and gasoline. When burned under the boilers in power plants, in home furnaces, in factories and in the engines of motor vehicles, fossil fuels give off five principal types of pollutants. Suspended particles include fly ash and other remnants of unburned fuel. Sulfur dioxide and nitrogen oxides, which are produced by the burning of coal and oil, can slowly mix with droplets of water to form highly corrosive sulfuric and nitric acids. Hydrocarbons and components of refined fuels like gasoline and diesel fuel are generally toxic and often carcinogenic. When fossil fuels are incompletely burned, for example in a furnace that needs adjustment, the result can be carbon monoxide, a compound that binds tightly to hemoglobin in red blood cells, lowering the ability of the body to get oxygen to its cells.

The compounds that exit from smokestacks and tailpipes are toxic enough by themselves, but many are transformed with the aid of sunlight to even more poisonous substances. The resulting photochemical smog is a deadly mixture of industrial-grade chemicals like formaldehyde and acrolein, a yellowish liquid that causes intense irritation to the lungs and eyes. One of the most common respiratory irritants in urban smog is created when nitrogen dioxide reacts with hydrocarbons and ultraviolet light and loses one of its two oxygen atoms. This lone atom can link with a normal molecule of oxygen to form a three-atom compound called ozone, a bluish gas with a characteristically pungent odor. In addition to being propagated in urban air, ozone is commonly created in the atmosphere around electrical devices. It is also the cause of the unpleasant smell near electric arcs, welding equipment, mercury-vapor lamps and photocopying machines.

Air Pollutants Move Indoors

Of the air pollution that exists within our houses, a small amount comes from the building materials used to make them. Formaldehyde, which causes nasal cancer in rodents, has been known to leach out of plywood and other building materials and, as we saw in Chapter 2, can be a severe problem in mobile homes. Radon gas is produced by bricks, cement and other materials made from stone and earth (more on radon gas below).

But we produce a great proportion of the fumes, particles and gases that drift through our homes ourselves. When we use spray cans, traces of the fluorocarbon propellants linger in the air. When we smoke cigarettes, the toxic effluent drifts around for hours. Fumes from cleaning products, pesticides from no-pest strips or bug sprays, and remnants of other common products are found in all homes. Since the levels of the toxic or carcinogenic compounds are often low, the health risk they pose is not known. But sometimes the concentrations can rise to dramatic levels. Within 90 minutes after a warm oven is sprayed with a commercial cleaner, levels of carcinogenic hydrocarbons can rise from near zero to 80 or 100 parts per million (Figure 1).

Figure 1
The Creation of Hydrocarbons by the Use of Oven Cleaner

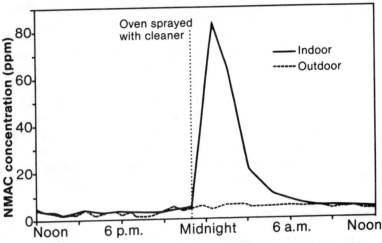

Activities in the home can have a profound effect on indoor air quality. In this case, the use of a commercial oven cleaner caused a marked rise in the concentration of a type of potentially carcinogenic substance known as nonmethane hydrocarbons (NMHC) in less than 90 minutes. Source: R. Whitaker, "Air Quality in the Home," *EPRI Journal*, March 1982.

In many buildings, particularly schools, offices and factories, there are tiny fibers of asbestos in the air. Asbestos is used in the making of ceiling tiles, vinyl floor tiles and a type of sprayed-on insulation. It was once widely used in public buildings and, in fact, building codes once required its installation in many buildings because of its fire-retardant characteristics. It is also used in cement water pipes, which accounts for its presence in many municipal water systems, and is found in brake linings, toasters, air conditioning systems and talcum powder.

In large amounts, asbestos fibers can cause a debilitating and sometimes fatal lung disease, known as asbestosis, as the fibers accumulate in the lungs and are not removed by normal biological processes. With time they can also cause lung cancer, particularly in industrial workers who also smoke, and have been linked with mesothelioma, an often fatal cancer of the chest and abdominal cavities. Whether ingested asbestos causes cancer in humans is unknown, but asbestos is of considerable concern to the EPA, given its presence at relatively high levels in many communities' drinking water.

If you work or attend school in a building built more than ten years ago, your chances of encountering asbestos are good. More recent buildings may also have an asbestos problem, as the mineral is still used in such products as floor tiles. Once thought to be an insignificant contributor to indoor asbestos pollution, floor tiles, which account for about 15 percent of United States asbestos production, were found to be a major source of deadly fibers in a recent study by three French scientists. They concluded that, in heavily trafficked areas, vinyl tiles that contain asbestos could contribute as much asbestos to the air as sprayed-on ceiling insulation.

In recent years, Americans have greatly increased the threat that indoor pollution poses by making the average home a much more efficient trap for pollutants. This trend began in 1973 when a cartel of foreign oil producers embargoed the supply of crude oil to the United States and grew stronger in 1978 with another major interruption in America's foreign oil pipeline. Oil prices soared, gas lines appeared and Americans began thinking seriously about conserving energy.

To save on heating costs, for example, many people weatherized their homes and started burning wood. The resulting energy savings have been significant. It would seem to be a happy ending, if it were not for the effect it is all having on human health. For example, insulating and weatherproofing homes tightens them up, allowing less circulation of air and trapping pollutants in the home. In addition, burning wood produces many toxins and at least a dozen cancer-causing agents. In our drive to make our homes efficient and energy-frugal, we have created a potentially catastrophic health problem.

Aside from ureaformaldehyde foam insulation, which leaches formaldehyde gas into the air, and sprayed-on asbestos, which can fill the air with asbestos fibers, insulation by itself generally poses no health risk. However, insulation, and especially weather-proofing, by design, cut down on the rate of air exchange between the house and the outside. While this reduces heat loss and slashes fuel bills, it also slows down the removal of pollutants from homes.

The Electric Power Research Institute (EPRI), a research organization supported by United States electric utilities, surveyed a number of homes and office buildings in Boston and found that the exchange rate varied from one complete turnover every 40 minutes to about one exchange every two hours. The better weatherproofed a home is, the longer the turnover time. New building materials and building methods may be able to decrease the exchange rate to once every five to ten hours.

Poor air circulation allows pollutants, such as hydrocarbon carcinogens from wood-burning or carbon monoxide from a gas range, to build up to unacceptable levels. In its Boston study, EPRI found that levels of nitrogen oxides and carbon monoxide were higher in all of the homes they examined than in the outside city air, no matter what type of heating was used. Levels of carbon monoxide peaked at five or more times the outdoor level around dinnertime in homes with gas ranges (Figure 2). Levels of particulate matter were also higher indoors, running from twice the outdoor level in some homes to 300 percent higher in houses where people smoked. The office buildings studied had better air quality than the homes because of their more efficient air conditioning and filtering systems.

One indoor air pollutant of particular concern to health scientists is radon gas. The product of the radioactive decay of radium, an element found in earthen building materials such as bricks, tiles, cinder blocks and concrete, radon gas is found in virtually all homes. Various surveys of homes and office buildings across the country have detected radon in every building sampled. There was little regional variation in radon levels. In fact, major

Figure 2
Creation of Carbon Monoxide in a Home Where Gas Is Used

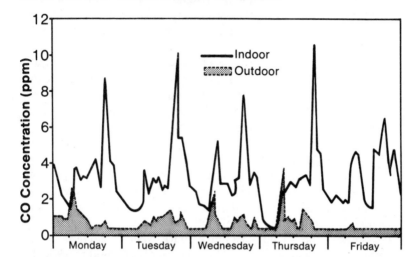

Levels of carbon monoxide (CO) in a house where natural gas is used frequently exceed outside CO levels, even in a city. The excess CO results from the burning of gas. Note in particular how CO level peaks sharply each day at dinnertime when the gas stove is on. Source: R. Whitaker, "Air Quality in the Home," *EPRI Journal,* March 1982.

differences in concentrations of the relatively short-lived gas can be attributed to differences in the amount of earthen materials in the homes and the rates of air exchange. Passive solar homes are generally the worst offenders. In addition to being very well-insulated, these homes incorporate a great deal of stone and concrete to store solar energy.

Radon gas is a potent carcinogen. When it becomes attached to the particles of dust that drift through every home, it can lodge in the lungs and cause cancer. Dr. Bernard Cohen of the University of Pittsburgh has estimated that exposure to radon gas now accounts for about 15,000 lung cancers in the United States each year. If the extensive weatherproofing programs envisioned by many regulators, government officials and utility executives are fully implemented, that figure could double. But, though faced with statistics like that, this nation need not question its commitment to conservation and energy independence. Instead, economical ways must be found to remove trapped pollutants and still retain precious heat. Unfortunately, most of the air exchange systems now on the market are too expensive for the average homeowner.

Weatherproofing is only one of the ways Americans have tried to save energy and money. Many homeowners, especially in the Northeast, which has a high reliance on imported oil, are turning back to wood for home heating. In the last ten years, the use of wood has risen dramatically. The Department of Energy's Energy Information Administration estimates that the total consumption of wood in the United States jumped 56 percent between 1970 and 1982. The number of homes using wood as their primary fuel for space heating doubled between 1979 and 1980 alone.

Currently, about five million homes use firewood as their main energy source. Another nine million use wood as a secondary heat source and an untold number burn wood in fireplaces. Together they consumed about 42 million cords of wood in 1980 (a cord is a stack of wood measuring four feet by four feet by eight feet or about 128 cubic feet). In addition, the Energy Department reports that the use of wood fuel by industry, primarily by lumber companies and paper mills, tripled between 1949 and 1981.

The crackle and warm glow of a wood fire on a cold night has become a symbol of the energy-conservation movement. As wholesome and old-fashioned as wood-burning may seem, it can pose a very serious health threat. Woodsmoke is laden with pollutants. Some, like heavy metals, are toxic, and others are known carcinogens.

One of the most-studied cancer-causing agents in woodsmoke is known as benzo(a)pyrene, or BaP. In the Boston homes monitored by the Electric Power Research Institute, benzo(a)pyrene, which seems to be produced in varying quantities when any organic material is burned, was present in levels about the same as or only slightly greater than outdoor city air. When a fireplace or woodstove was operating, however, the concentration climbed to several times outdoor levels (Figure 3).

Just as woodstoves and fireplaces are enjoying a renascence,

Figure 3
Relationship Between Woodburning and Benzo(a)pyrene Concentration

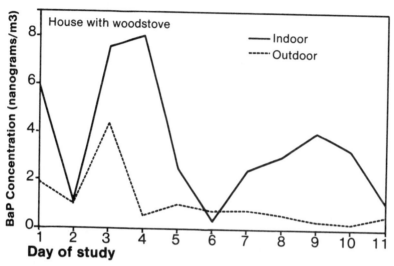

In this house, where a woodstove is used for heating, levels of benzo(a)-pyrene, or BaP, a known carcinogen, were considerably higher indoors than outdoors every day the stove was in use. The stove was not fired up on days 2, 6 or 11. Source: R. Whitaker, "Air Quality in the Home," *EPRI Journal*, March 1982.

the once popular kerosene heater is coming back into style. But, as with woodstoves, kerosene heaters have brought with them an important public health threat. The safety of unvented, portable kerosene heaters came into question in 1982 when the Consumers Union, publishers of *Consumer Reports*, claimed their tests showed that the normal use of these heaters could result in hazardous levels of several air pollutants. The findings of Consumers Union were confirmed by the Consumer Product Safety Commission later that year and by independent researchers.

For example, in December of 1982, Dr. Brian P. Leaderer of Yale University's Department of Epidemiology and Public Health published in *Science* the results of tests in which he ran kerosene heaters in a 12-foot by 12-foot by 8-foot chamber that simulated a room in a house. He found that convective and radiant kerosene heaters, both normally used without any ventilation, produced levels of nitrogen dioxide and sulfur dioxide that exceeded federal standards for outdoor air. In addition, he found that concentrations of carbon dioxide exceeded occupational health standards. Levels of hydrocarbons, Leaderer found, tended to rise only after the heaters were turned off, apparently generated by the still-warm wick.

Fighting Air Pollutants with Diet

The air at times seems thick with pollutants and charged with toxins that harm the lungs, interfere with the ability of our blood to carry oxygen or alter the genetic makeup of our cells. Unfortunately, the literature of public health science is not equally thick with research on nutritional interactions with these pollutants. Of the pollutants we have mentioned in this section, only three types have been even moderately well-studied. These are the respiratory irritants ozone and nitrogen dioxide; ionizing radiation, such as that emitted by radon gas; and the hydrocarbon carcinogen benzo(a)pyrene. Many other important pollutants, such as carbon monoxide and asbestos, have been studied only superficially, if at all. Here is the most reliable information we now have on the interaction between air pollution and diet.

OZONE AND NITROGEN DIOXIDE: When ozone or nitrogen dioxide contacts the lining of the respiratory tract, it snatches electrons from the biological molecules that make up the lining of the throat, trachea, bronchial passages and lungs. This is a process scientists call oxidation, in recognition of the ability of oxygen to react with other compounds and remove electrons.

The molecules that ozone and nitrogen dioxide oxidize are called unsaturated lipids, and they make up the outer layers of cell membranes. When these lipids become oxidized, the membranes of the cells in the respiratory tract are weakened. The result can range from a dry, scratchy throat to pulmonary edema, an accumulation of fluids in the respiratory tissue. Prolonged exposure to ozone can cause headaches, drowsiness and a slowing of the heart and breathing rates. Both ozone and nitrogen dioxide also seem able to speed the aging of lung and skin tissues. The elderly and sufferers of respiratory ailments are most likely to become ill. But it is not just the infirm or the aged who fall victim to airborne oxidizing agents. Evidence from several studies suggests that vigorous exercise enhances the effects of ozone and nitrogen dioxide on the lungs and other physiological systems. One study found that the performance of high-school cross-country runners deteriorated as the level of ozone in the air rose. Other athletes have been affected in the same way. When athletes exercise, their respiration rates increase and they breathe air deeper into the lungs, where it comes into more intimate contact with the respiratory tissue. In addition, heavy exertion tends to switch breathing from the nose to the mouth. Unlike the nose, the mouth is unable to filter out pollutants.

One way to reduce the damage caused by oxidants such as ozone is with antioxidants, which combine with oxidants and disarm them. Two common antioxidants, vitamin C and vitamin E, are found in food. Research with both of these nutrients has confirmed their ability to protect the body from respiratory irritants.

Vitamin C seems to work by capturing oxidants such as ozone and nitrogen dioxide or their by-products before they reach sensitive tissue in the respiratory tract. The vitamin latches on to them in the fluid that bathes the tissue of the air passages and lungs, inactivating the molecules and preventing them from crossing into the bloodstream. In work with rats, supplements of vitamin C have lowered the death rate from and the occurrence of pulmonary edema in animals exposed to extraordinarily large doses of ozone. Vitamin C also seems to act as a natural antihistamine, deactivating the histamine that is produced when the lungs are irritated and that may be responsible for the pulmonary edema that follows a heavy dose of ozone. Unfortunately, it is not yet possible to estimate from the animal studies how much vitamin C the human body requires to offset the effects of ozone exposure. In addition, it is not yet known to what extent a deficiency of vitamin C changes one's susceptibility to lower, more commonly encountered levels of ozone and other oxidants.

Unsaturated fats are a prime component of the membranes of the cells that line the respiratory tract, and they are believed to be particularly susceptible to the oxidizing effects of ozone and nitrogen dioxide. Since vitamin E is known to protect fats from oxidation, scientists have studied the effects of supplements of vitamin E on oxidant-induced lung damage.

In a 1979 study, rats were fed diets either deficient in or supplemented with vitamin E and then exposed to a moderate dose of nitrogen dioxide. The rats on the supplemented diet suffered far less damage to the lipids in their respiratory tract. In another study, researchers examined the amount of time required for half of a group of rats exposed to one part per million of ozone to die when fed varying diets. Rats fed a vitamin E deficient diet developed edema more rapidly and died twice as quickly as those on an adequate diet.

Of great significance was the fact that tissue damage occurred at ozone levels only slightly greater than those commonly found in city air. Since this implies that ozone and nitrogen dioxide probably pose a serious health risk to many people, particularly the elderly, the infirm and athletes, the question arises as to how much vitamin E we need to consume to protect our lungs from these pollutants. According to a 1973 report by B. L. Fletcher and A. L. Tappel, 30 milligrams of vitamin E per day is probably adequate to put up a good defense. However, the average adult intake is only one-quarter of this amount.

In addition to its effects on respiratory tissue, ozone and its byproducts can also cause toxic reactions in the body. In animal tests, ozone has been found to produce abnormal chromosomes in white blood cells and granular particles in red blood cells that indicate damage to the hemoglobin molecule. Studying the red blood cells of human volunteers, Dr. Daniel Menzel and his colleagues at Duke University in 1975 found that giving human volunteers vitamin E supplements could prevent the formation of these particles after exposure to a toxic by-product of ozone.

IONIZING RADIATION: Little research has been done to determine how diet affects the reaction of the body to ionizing radiation, such as that given off by radon gas in the home. Limited work with animals suggests that vitamin A may protect against skin damage from very large radiation doses. In addition, an adequate amount of protein in the diet seems necessary to reduce the toxicity of radiation, and sulfur-containing amino acids may offer some protection as well. Large doses of vitamin C can reduce the gross effects of large radiation doses in test animals. Unfortunately, none of this research addresses the effects of nutrition on smaller, more realistic radiation levels or determines the ability of nutrition to cut down the human risk of cancer induced by radiation.

BENZO(A)PYRENE: Some work has been done on benzo(a)pyrene and its chemical carcinogen cousins. A growing body of research has attempted to determine what effect a deficiency or supplement of the B vitamin riboflavin has on benzo(a)pyrene, but with mixed results. The most encouraging research concerns the ability of vitamin A to reduce the occurrence of benzo(a)pyrene-induced cancer (see the smoking section of Chapter 9). Much more work needs to be done in these areas, especially in light of the increasing popularity of wood-burning. The food additives BHT and BHA may also prove useful in preventing the carcinogenic effects of benzo(a)pyrene. See Chapter 5 for more on this interaction.

Thus, we can say that while the data available on nutritional interactions with benzo(a)pyrene and radiation are disappointingly sketchy, the story is somewhat better for the common respiratory irritants ozone and nitrogen dioxide. It appears that vitamin A and the food additives BHT and BHA may offer some protection against benzo(a)pyrene, but a great deal of work is still needed to confirm this. On the other hand, it has been proved in animal tests that vitamin E reduces the amount of damage that ozone and nitrogen dioxide can do to the respiratory tract. Although it is too early to make strong recommendations, it would appear that anyone routinely exposed to ozone or nitrogen dioxide should be careful to eat a diet rich in vitamin E (see Chapter 3 for some suggested sources). In particular, the elderly and athletes, who are at a heightened risk to respiratory irritants, should bolster their consumption of vitamin E.

CONCLUSION: NUTRITION AND
THE PERILS AROUND US

Despite our best efforts and the best-intentioned plans of government and industry, we will never have a pollution-free world. Our daily lives will continue to be spent in a sea of chemical compounds that threaten our health and lives. Lead in the air, soil and water has already had a tragic effect on the health and mental capabilities of millions of children. Cadmium and organic chemicals are ubiquitous in our drinking water and food and steadily accumulate in our tissues. Ozone, nitrogen oxides, radon gas and carcinogens like benzo(a)pyrene pollute the air outside and inside our homes and workplaces.

At the beginning of this chapter we noted that many people believe that nutrition may help protect them against the various insults in the environment. Just how valid are these beliefs? Can the right diet lower one's susceptibility to the pollutants in the world around us? Can vitamins, minerals and other nutrients provide a shield against environmental disease?

On the whole, the answer to those questions seems to be probably. To date the evidence is promising, but not nearly conclusive. The majority of work examining nutritional interactions with common air, water and household pollutants has been done with laboratory animals. For example, by working with animals we know:

—That the minerals calcium, phosphorus, copper, magnesium and iron, as well as vitamins C and E and apple pectin, seem able to markedly lower the toxicity of the pervasive heavy metal lead.

—That zinc, iron, calcium and vitamin C can prevent or lessen many of the toxic effects of cadmium.

—That vitamin A and the synthetic antioxidants BHA and BHT may block the cancer-causing ability of the wood-smoke pollutant benzo(a)pyrene.

—And that vitamin E is very effective in reducing the damage ozone and nitrogen dioxide can do to the lining of the respiratory tract.

While animals can serve as excellent models of the human response to the environment, a great deal more work with people still needs to be done before many firm conclusions can be drawn. Meanwhile, as we noted above, it seems safe to say that in some cases nutrition does offer the human body a degree of security from common environmental pollutants. But exactly how much protection these nutrients afford and at what doses is still uncertain.

For some pollutants, most notably carbon monoxide, formaldehyde, asbestos, sulfur dioxide and a slew of organic chemicals, there are few known nutrient interactions. In some cases, relatively little or no work has been done to date to evaluate the effects of nutrition on these pollutants. In others, no effects have yet turned up.

As with pollutants in food, there is great promise that nutrition may one day prove to be one effective way to lower our risk from the environment. The groundwork has been laid. What is needed now is a comprehensive effort to understand just how great a role diet can play.

CHAPTER 7

Occupational Hazards: The Chemicals We Work With

There are more than 70,000 chemical compounds being manufactured in the United States today. Each year another 700 to 3,000 new substances are added to that list. While many are relatively nontoxic, others cause adverse effects on the body that range from skin irritations to cancer.

Although many of these chemicals ultimately reach the environment, they are not hazards only as environmental pollutants. They pose a very real danger to the millions of people who work in manufacturing plants where these substances are made, in factories where they are used to make other products and in businesses and homes where those products are ultimately used. For many reasons, workers who make and work directly with these chemicals are at the greatest risk. They are more likely to be exposed to high and potentially dangerous levels of these chemicals.

Spurred largely by government regulations, manufacturers and industries have attempted to protect workers from exposure to harmful substances or conditions. Work areas have been better ventilated; handling and processing techniques improved to reduce the escape of toxic fumes and dust; and workers provided with breathing apparatus, air filters and protective clothing. But, even with these measures, contact with dangerous chemicals cannot be eliminated.

One potential weapon against chemical toxins and carcinogens that has been largely ignored by government and industry is nutritional supplementation. This chapter evaluates the evidence that the adverse effects of many industrial chemicals can be prevented or alleviated to a significant extent with normal or larger-than-normal amounts of nutrients, and aggravated by marginally adequate diets. We will discuss nearly 20 compounds in the following pages, so to avoid greatly lengthening the chapter we have left all our recommendations for the conclusion of this chapter.

INORGANIC CHEMICALS

Arsenic

Long the poison of choice among villains in murder mysteries, arsenic, a highly toxic metal, is used widely in industry. Metal workers, drug producers, gold refiners, insecticide makers, lead smelters, painters, taxidermists, petroleum refinery workers, tree sprayers and workers in many other industries may be exposed to arsenic.

Frequent contact with arsenic can burn or redden the skin. A small number of skin cancers among industrial workers have also been linked to arsenic. A worker exposed to an excessive dose of arsenic, usually inhaled as dust, will first complain of weakness, loss of appetite, nausea, diarrhea and occasional vomiting. If the symptoms persist, the worker may experience inflammation of the eyes, nose, nerves and respiratory tract and a perforated nasal septum (the partition that separates the nostrils), as well as paralysis of the muscles in the toes. Cases of severe or fatal arsenic poisoning are rare in industry, but workers do occasionally suffer from chronic poisoning.

Although the dangers of arsenic had been known for many years, its potency was demonstrated inadvertently between 1925 and 1939 when the United States Navy Medical Corps treated cases of syphilis with a drug that contained an arsenic compound known as neoarsphenamine. Over one million doses of the drug were administered during those 14 years, and for every 4,000 doses, there was one death or severe reaction. Many other patients experienced milder side effects.

Subsequent research showed that the symptoms of acute arsenic poisoning suffered by those who took the drug (no longer in use) could be reversed or prevented with high doses of vitamin C. In fact, those most susceptible to the negative effects of the drug were persons with a vitamin C deficiency. Diets high in protein or carbohydrates, especially diets of low-fat meats, have also been found to reduce the severity of reactions to arsenical drugs. Whether such diets will also help industrial workers exposed to arsenic has yet to be tested.

Chromium

Chromium, the shiny metal that graces automobile bumpers, is used in several occupations. Copper etchers, glass blowers, welders, photoengravers, textile workers and lithographers are all likely to come into contact with it.

When chromium touches the skin, it can cause a type of inflammation known as dermatitis. When it is ingested or inhaled, chromium can induce coughing, headaches, painful breathing, fever and loss of weight. Some workers, especially those in the electroplating business, may suffer more severe symptoms, such as swelling of the eyes and chronic asthma and bronchitis. Acids containing chromium may cause cancer, and several studies have found a high incidence of lung cancer among workers who handle chromium ore.

The danger from chromium compounds is related to a property of chemicals known as valence. Valence refers to the ability of an atom to combine with other atoms. Each element is assigned a valence number, which is an indication of how many atoms of hydrogen (the simplest of atoms) it can link with. The chromium compounds that have a valence number of three seem to be relatively inert, primarily causing occasional allergic reactions. The most serious health hazards are associated with compounds that have a valence of six. It is not surprising that a great deal of research has been devoted to finding ways to convert the six-valent, or hexavalent, compounds to the less harmful trivalent forms. One naturally occurring chemical that can catalyze this transformation is vitamin C.

When mixed in the laboratory, one gram of ascorbic acid will convert a little over a tenth of a gram of hexavalent chromium to trivalent chromium. Vitamin C also seems to be able to repair the damage done by hexavalent chromium. When vitamin C is applied to ulcers on the skin of guinea pigs treated with chromium, the ulcers heal much more quickly than ulcers that are not treated in this way.

In experimental trials, the incidence and severity of skin ulcers and other skin problems in industrial workers has been drastically reduced when the workers were encouraged to quickly wash contaminated skin with a ten-percent solution of vitamin C. Nose ulcers have also been prevented by passing air from the workplace through filters impregnated with ascorbic acid.

Silica and Quartz Dust

Vitamin C can also alleviate a degenerative lung disease caused by inhaling silica and quartz dust. Called silicosis, the condition is characterized by lumps or nodules in the lung tissue. In severe cases, the nodules can develop into scar tissue and lead to emphysema. Silicosis is a threat primarily in such occupations as construction, cement manufacturing, stone-cutting and gravel-quarrying.

Because it can help heal wounds, vitamin C has been tested for its ability to prevent and cure silicosis. In studies with rats, vitamin C slowed the formation of scar tissue after exposure to silica dust. Guinea pigs made to breathe in silica dust seemed to concentrate ascorbic acid in their lung tissue in an apparent attempt to head off tissue damage. Whether vitamin C supplements can counter the onset of silicosis in humans remains to be tested.

Silver

Hearing the word silver brings to mind images of jewelry and silverware. But silver is quite useful in industry as well. Alloys of silver are found in coins, Christmas tree ornaments, scientific instruments, printed circuits and automobile bearings. Silver is used in the manufacture of bactericides, photographic chemicals, drugs, dental fillings, hair dyes, glass, solder, mirrors, ceramics and electrical equipment, and is also used by ivory etchers and in water treatment.

Silver is not a highly toxic metal, but long-term exposure to the skin, digestive tract or lungs can cause a condition known as argyria. Sufferers of this affliction have a blue-gray discoloration of the skin, eyes and mucous membranes. Although silver must usually enter the body to cause argyria, workers who get bits of silver implanted in their skin or nasal passages may notice a permanent staining.

In rare cases, exposure to silver can also cause kidney, liver and spleen damage. Work with rats has shown that animals fed a diet deficient in vitamin E and exposed to silver are much more likely to suffer tissue damage than rats fed a normal diet. In fact, when deficient rats were given a vitamin E supplement, the damage often cleared up. The vitamin deficiency seemed to make the rats particularly susceptible to liver damage, something that should be taken into consideration by companies that use silver, since vitamin E deficiencies are fairly common.

Tellurium

The element tellurium, used primarily in the vulcanization of rubber, is unusual in that the principal risk it poses to industrial workers is not one of health, but of social acceptance. Anyone who has seen too many mouthwash commercials can sympathize with the plight of the worker who has been exposed to a large dose of tellurium or to smaller doses over a long period of time. Tellurium makes the breath and perspiration smell strongly of garlic.

Fortunately, treatment with vitamin C can eliminate or greatly reduce the offensive breath. Apparently, vitamin C prevents the conversion of tellurium to the foul-smelling substance that plagues tellurium workers.

Vanadium

Workers who clean out the insides of boilers fired with oil often experience a variety of respiratory ills within a few hours or days after emerging from their sooty workplace. The symptoms include bloody noses, sore throats, coughing, inflamed windpipes and bronchitis. Workers often suffer repeated bouts of bronchitis, even after they no longer go into the boilers.

The culprit is vanadium, a white or gray lustrous metallic element used in the making of special steels. As with chromium, treatment with vitamin C has dramatically reduced the effects of vanadium in laboratory animals. In one early study, excess vitamin C in the diet offered protection against amounts of vanadium that would otherwise nearly always prove fatal. In other work with rats, dogs and chickens, vitamin C proved effective if administered in large doses and injected shortly after the administration of vanadium.

Unfortunately, the levels of vitamin C used in this research were much higher than normal human consumption. Also, the vanadium used in the experiments was either fed to or injected into the test animals, while the principal route of exposure for people is airborne vanadium. However, the evidence to date at least suggests that vitamin C could curb vanadium toxicity in boiler workers.

Thallium

Used widely in industry, thallium is a highly toxic and long-acting poison. It is, in fact, one of the most toxic elements known. A case of thallium poisoning can start with fatigue, limb pain, a metallic taste in the mouth and the loss of hair. More severe cases are characterized by eye damage, gastrointestinal distress, colic, impaired kidney function, neuritis, convulsions and disorientation.

There have been many known cases of fatal thallium poisoning. Many of these involved children who ingested pesticides laden with this toxic substance. Thallium can also be a hazard to artificial diamond makers, manufacturers of photoelectric cells, glass makers, fireworks manufacturers, optical glass fashioners, dye makers and pesticide workers.

That nutrition might alter the toxicity of thallium was first suggested in the 1940s when it was observed that the type of fodder eaten by sheep determined how they would react to exposure to thallium and that brewer's yeast could prevent the cataracts and loss of hair that thallium is known to cause. Brewer's yeast was apparently supplying the sheep with an amino acid known as cystine. Thallium seems to prevent the body from manufacturing enough cystine, causing the deficiency symptoms seen in thallium poisoning. Whether cystine supplements will be effective in preventing thallium poisoning in people has not been adequately tested.

ORGANIC COMPOUNDS

Benzene Derivatives

In the latter half of the nineteenth century, a German chemist, Friedrich August Kekule von Stradonitz, was struggling to determine the structure of a molecule known as benzene. Kekule knew that the molecule had six atoms of carbon and six atoms of hydrogen, and he knew some of its unusual properties. But he could not come up with a shape that would make sense of this compound.

One evening he had a dream. He saw the six carbon atoms of benzene dancing in a circle, holding hands. From this image, he deduced that the benzene molecule is a ring of carbon atoms. With this revelation, Kekule unwittingly opened up a highly important and fruitful branch of organic chemistry.

Benzene and the many compounds that can be made by attaching other atoms to the six-carbon benzene ring have found numerous uses in industry. Known collectively as aromatic compounds because of their strong and usually pleasant odors, they include naphthalene, found in mothballs; styrene, which can be made into the common plastic polystyrene; toluene, a solvent found in paint thinner and a useful chemical building block; and xylene, a versatile compound employed in the making of adhesives, inks, dyes, perfumes, insect repellents, epoxy resins and pharmaceuticals.

One characteristic many aromatics have in common is an unusually high toxicity. They often are capable of causing nervous system damage and destroying the tissues of the liver, kidneys and bone marrow. Many benzene derivatives are also carcinogenic. This was first discovered in the early part of this century when workers who handled coal tar, a gooey black material created when bituminous coal is heated in the absence of air, were found to have an unusually high incidence of skin cancer. The cancers were similar to those that had been seen in English chimney sweeps since the late nineteenth century. It was later learned that the cause of the cancers was certain aromatic compounds in coal tar, including benzo(a)pyrene, a component of cigarette smoke.

Although many benzene derivatives are known to cause cancer, the cancer-inducing ability of benzene itself, the simplest of the aromatics, is still in question, though it is believed to cause leukemia, a cancer in which the white blood cells, or leukocytes, multiply uncontrollably. Even if benzene were not a carcinogen, it would still be considered a hazardous chemical, since it can do severe damage to the tissues that manufacture white blood cells. Abnormally developed bone marrow, a high number of white cells in the blood and an abnormally low number of granular leukocytes (a class of white blood cells involved in fighting off infections and in the allergic response) are all signs of the type of tissue damage benzene causes.

The mineral selenium can prevent the destruction of the blood-forming organs by benzene. In one study, when given to rats for ten days prior to exposure to benzene, selenium prevented or markedly retarded some of the toxic effects of this organic solvent. Several other experiments have yielded similar findings. These results are encouraging enough for some scientists to suggest that selenium may be able to prevent leukemia or leukemialike symptoms in industrial workers exposed to benzene.

While selenium's role in preventing benzene-induced tissue damage is still speculative, the ability of vitamin C, perhaps in larger-than-normal amounts, to protect the body from benzene is well known. The connection between benzene poisoning and vitamin C was first suspected when it was noticed that one of the symptoms of benzene intoxication, bleeding from the skin and mucous membranes, is similar to a manifestation of scurvy or a severe vitamin C deficiency.

Unfortunately, much of the work in this area has been marred by inadequate experimental design or controls, but at least one important study was free of flaws. In 1947, two researchers found that workers in a rotogravure printing shop who breathed in benzene while on the job took a few days longer to produce urine saturated with vitamin C after ingesting vitamin supplements than coworkers who were not regularly exposed to the chemical. From this, the researchers concluded that the exposed workers were using up more vitamin C than nonexposed workers, presumably to fight off benzene. When this theory was tested in a South African chemical plant, workers avoided benzene poisoning simply by drinking orange juice every day.

In addition to drinking orange juice, benzene-exposed workers should also consume a diet that contains at least the recommended daily intake of protein. Protein seems to help detoxify benzene. It is believed that sulfur-containing amino acids in protein are responsible for this effect. Too much fat in the diet, on the other hand, markedly increases one's chances of being poisoned by benzene.

Carbon Tetrachloride

This is a colorless liquid used in fire extinguishers, as a solvent and cleaning agent and in a number of industrial applications. Although frequent contact with the skin can cause a scaly form of dermatitis, the main danger to industrial workers comes from inhaling carbon tetrachloride vapors. In the body, carbon tetrachloride can depress the central nervous system and damage the liver and kidneys. The effects are enhanced by alcohol and fats, both of which step up the intestinal absorption of carbon tetrachloride.

The liver is the organ most seriously damaged by this chemical. Affected workers often develop jaundice and excrete red and white blood cells in their urine. In animal tests, carbon tetrachloride has also been found to cause liver cancer. No thorough evaluation of the cancer risk posed by exposure of industrial workers to carbon tetrachloride has been undertaken, but it is reasonable to assume that the severe liver damage the compound can cause may lead to cancers in some cases.

Two B vitamins, B_{12} and nicotinic acid, may offer some protection against the liver damage and possible liver cancers caused by carbon tetrachloride. However, in animal studies, the vitamins were effective only if administered in large doses before exposure to the chemical. Doses given after the animals were injected with carbon tetrachloride were of little help. Part of the beneficial action of B_{12} may stem from the vitamin's role in helping the body use protein. In animal studies, protein has proved effective in preventing or reducing damage done by carbon tetrachloride. There is evidence that the active agent may again not be protein itself, but sulfur-containing amino acids. The sulfur in one amino acid in particular, methionine, seems to protect and heal the liver.

Vinyl Chloride

In December 1973 a worker at a B. F. Goodrich chemical plant in Louisville, Kentucky, died from a rare form of liver cancer. Known as angiosarcoma, this type of tumor can be expected to turn up in only 25 to 30 Americans in an average year. But this was the third death from angiosarcoma at the Louisville plant in three and a half years. An obvious culprit for the cancers was the chemical the three workers had handled, vinyl chloride. A link was established between the chemical and cancer when a check showed that angiosarcoma had been the cause of a number of other deaths at vinyl chloride plants elsewhere.

Vinyl chloride, a colorless liquid when cooled and a flammable gas that smells like ether at room temperature, is a simple organic molecule that can be linked into long chains to form the plastic polyvinyl chloride, or PVC. In addition to inducing cancer, vinyl chloride can cause the bones in the tips of the fingers to deteriorate and the skin to turn alternately bluish or pale and inflamed. There is also evidence that this compound can seriously damage the liver, even in workers who do not ultimately get liver cancer. Vinyl chloride seems to be toxic and carcinogenic only at fairly high doses. The workers who developed cancer were regularly exposed to concentrations of 1,000 to several thousand parts per million.

To date, only one study suggesting that nutrition can protect against vinyl chloride toxicity has been conducted, but the results were encouraging. In the study, published in 1975, guinea pigs were subjected to vinyl chloride and fed a diet that included a daily supplement of ten milligrams of vitamin C (about the amount in two orange segments). Damage to the liver and kidneys was reduced with the vitamin C treatment.

Conditions in vinyl chloride plants have improved dramatically in recent years and workers are less likely to be exposed to large amounts of the chemical. Even so, the limited evidence suggests that workers should eat foods rich in vitamin C every day.

Chloroform

Once used widely as an anesthetic, chloroform is now found primarily in industry. This colorless liquid is used in the manufacture of penicillin and other drugs, in the production of artificial silk and in the making of floor waxes and plastics. The same characteristics that ultimately reduced chloroform's popularity as an anesthetic also make it a danger in the workplace. Exposure to large amounts of chloroform can badly damage the liver and kidneys. There is also conclusive evidence from studies done by the National Cancer Institute with mice and rats that it causes liver and kidney cancer, respectively.

Dietary intakes of proteins, fats and carbohydrates all affect the body's susceptibility to chloroform-induced damage. Both protein and carbohydrates offer some protection, especially when eaten in excess of normal requirements. High levels of fat, on the other hand, seem to cause the liver to concentrate chloroform, greatly increasing the amount of damage it can do. Although these findings are of particular importance to industrial workers, their significance may be more widespread.

When drinking water that contains a high level of organic material (for example, water from a reservoir with a bottom covered by decaying leaves) is disinfected with chlorine, one of the by-products of the chlorination process is often chloroform. In small amounts, chloroform flows out of the tap in millions of homes across the United States. In a 1975 survey of water supplies around the nation, the United States Environmental Protection Agency detected chloroform in nearly 100 percent of the supplies tested.

The significance of this is being hotly debated by scientists in the field of public health. By conducting lifetime tests with animals, these scientists have estimated that drinking two liters of water containing ten parts per billion of chloroform every day would be expected to cause cancer in about 100 people nationwide each year. In fact, chloroform levels as high as 366 parts per billion have been detected in United States drinking water. The prevalence of high-fat diets among Americans makes these projections particularly alarming, in light of the ability of fat to enhance chloroform damage to the liver.

TNT (Trinitrotoluene)

With the growing national concern about nuclear arms, it is easy to forget that our national defense is still built on a foundation of conventional weapons. These include—as they have for decades— bombs, shells, mines and other explosive devices. Since the dough-boys went to battle in World War I, one of the prime ingredients in these deadly packages has been a chemical known as trinitro-toluene, or TNT. TNT is also a commonly used explosive in the demolition business. Thus, between civilian and military orders, the national munitions industry is kept busy.

It has long been known that workers in this industry are subject to a variety of ills. TNT can irritate the eyes, nose and throat and stain the skin, hair and nails yellow. If ingested, it can cause death by severe hepatitis or a severe anemia resulting from destruction of the bone marrow. Repeated exposure to TNT can cause muscle pains, irregularities in the heartbeat, kidney irritations, cataracts, abnormal menstrual cycles, neuritis and methemoglobinemia, a condition in which red blood cells are rendered unable to carry oxygen to the body's cells.

The first indications that nutrition might offer some protection against these symptoms appeared during World War I. To support the United States war effort, production of TNT had been stepped up. As the output of the explosive rose, so did reports of toxic reactions. In one large munitions plant, the manager noticed that women seemed to suffer stomach upsets more often than the men. Suspecting that this difference might be due to the women's generally poorer nutrition, the manager started a program to improve the women's diet. In only four months, the proportion of women reporting stomach problems dropped from nearly 12 percent to under 1 percent.

Since then, nutrition programs have been common in the explosives industry. Although most of these programs have concentrated on a general improvement in nutrition among workers, there is evidence that a few nutrients are better than others in the fight against TNT. One is vitamin C.

As long ago as 1927, it was observed that some of the symptoms of TNT toxicity resembled those of scurvy. Studies with animals since then have shown that vitamin C, in greater-than-required amounts, does offer at least some protection against TNT. Vitamin C has proved useful in modifying the negative effects of TNT on red blood cells, especially in the cat and other animals that are particularly susceptible to this effect. How well vitamin C will protect people is not known.

1,2-Dichloroethane and 1,2-Dichloropropane

Although these compounds are not exactly household names, they are used extensively in industry and were probably involved in the manufacture of many things in your home. The plastic polyvinyl chloride, the synthetic fabrics nylon and rayon, rubber and certain paints are all made with the aid of 1,2-dichloroethane. It is also used in photography, xerography, and water-softening and in the manufacture of adhesives, cosmetics and medications. In addition, it serves as a dry-cleaning agent, a fumigant and an antiknock additive in gasoline. The chemically similar 1,2-dichloropropane is also used as a fumigant and dry-cleaning product and has proved useful in the making of waxes, scouring compounds, metal degreasers, paints and cellulose.

Both of these chemicals can damage the liver and kidneys. The susceptibility of laboratory animals to such effects is enhanced by deficiencies of protein, certain amino acids and the B vitamin choline. Supplementing the diet with the amino acid methionine offered some protection against 1,000 parts per million of either compound (13 times the federal standard for 1,2-dichloropropane and 20 times the limit for 1,2-dichloroethane). Methionine was able to reduce the mortality rate of laboratory animals from 100 percent to 10 percent in one study.

Carbon Disulfide

Carbon disulfide is used to make products as diverse as rubber cement and rocket fuel. Rayon, rubber, solvents and pesticides are all produced with the aid of this compound. Prolonged exposure to carbon disulfide can cause irritability, manic-depressive tendencies, headaches and neuritis (an inflammation of the nerves). By damaging the sheaths around nerve cells, it can disrupt the senses of sight and smell. In some cases, it has contributed to the development of atherosclerosis and coronary heart disease and it can cause chronic inflammation of the stomach and persistent menstrual disorders.

The B vitamins nicotinic acid and pyridoxine can prevent some of this damage when consumed at levels equal to or larger than the RDA, while deficiencies of either vitamin increase the body's susceptibility to carbon disulfide. In particular, nicotinic acid can prevent atherosclerosis in exposed animals. Some of the psychological disorders associated with carbon disulfide exposure can be relieved with pyridoxine. In fact, physicians have used this vitamin to successfully treat these symptoms.

Tricresyl Phosphate

To make certain plastics soft and pliable, manufacturers add plasticizers. One plasticizer, used in the production of polystyrene, vinyl and polyacrylics, is called tricresyl phosphate. When absorbed through the skin, inhaled or swallowed, this compound damages cells in the spinal cord and can also induce vomiting, diarrhea and abdominal pain.

A diet high in protein may prevent most of the toxic effects of tricresyl phosphate, the results of a 1953 study indicated. Vitamin E may also offer some protection, although not as effectively as protein. Unfortunately, no follow-up studies to expand these findings, including work with human subjects, has been attempted.

NOISE

Loud, distracting and nerve-racking noise is a common problem in modern industry. The bustling machinery of an assembly line, the roar of jet engines, the rumble of construction equipment, the din of a power plant, the pounding of a jackhammer, the whine of saws and cutting tools and the boom of a pile driver are all signs of progress, but they are also potential causes of hearing impairment and a host of psychological problems.

Loud noises can cause temporary or permanent hearing loss, depending on the intensity of the sound, the pitch, the duration of exposure and the individual's resistance to loud sounds. For many, exposure to just a few hours of sound with an intensity of 100 decibels can produce a troubling though short-lived loss of hearing. This is equivalent to the din in a kitchen in which a blender, dishwasher and mixer are all running simultaneously and is somewhat quieter than a loud rock band. It is also greater than the federal limit on noise in the workplace. Sound at this level heard day after day may cause permanent deafness.

Loud noises can also raise blood pressure and cause sweating and twitching muscles. These are elements of the so-called fight-or-flight reaction to stress. It is useful when one is faced with real danger, but it can be destructive when triggered day after day with no physical release.

There is evidence that vitamins A and C may soften the effects of loud noise. In the 1940s and 1950s, scientists were able to successfully treat tinnitus, a ringing in the ear, with vitamin A. Auditory fatigue, a form of temporary hearing loss, also responded to the vitamin treatment. From this and later work it has become clear that vitamin A can prevent hearing loss, but only at levels that are so high as to be poisonous to other parts of the body.

More promising findings have been obtained from research with vitamin C. Two studies done in the 1960s at a Moscow brake factory provide the best evidence to date that vitamin C may prevent hearing loss. Six workers received 100 milligrams of vitamin C (about twice the recommended daily adult dose) each day after lunch while a control group was given a placebo. The workers who received the vitamin were rated better at muscle endurance and fatigue (two factors that are affected by noise) than the control group. Unfortunately, the researchers did not check to see if the tested workers smoked or had other habits that could affect the body burden of vitamin C. The final word on this subject, therefore, must await further study.

CONCLUSIONS: SAFETY IN THE LUNCH BUCKET

In an ideal world, all industrial workers would labor in a clean, safe environment. But the world is not ideal and the industrial environment is too often contaminated with fumes, dust, noise and other hazards. Government regulations and public pressure have gone a long way toward improving conditions in many industries. The level of vinyl chloride fumes in plants that manufacture that plastic building block, for example, dropped considerably after the chemical was linked to cancer.

But the cost of offering complete protection to workers is often prohibitive, so industry and government compromise and set standards that industry can meet and that offer a reasonable amount of protection for workers. By setting standards, one does not eliminate occupational exposure to hazardous chemicals. Workers will still face hazards in the workplace and many may become sick. A smaller number will likely die as a result of their jobs.

As this chapter has pointed out, a largely unexplored but potentially significant safeguard for industrial workers is nutrition. Supplements of vitamins, minerals and other nutrients have proven effective in studies with both animals and humans in preventing or at least reducing the negative health effects of common industrial chemicals. Supplements of vitamin C can prevent at least some of the adverse effects of arsenic, chromium, silica, tellurium, benzene and other chemicals. In particular, vitamin C has proved useful in preventing or alleviating skin and nose ulcers from topical exposure to chromium, may alleviate a debilitating lung disease known as silicosis that results from exposure to silica and quartz dust and has reduced the internal, though not the respiratory, effects of exposure to vanadium.

Other work has shown that protein consumed at normal or higher-than-normal levels seems to protect the body against benzene, chloroform, carbon tetrachloride and tricresyl phosphate toxicity. It is probably not protein itself but the sulfur-containing amino acids the protein contains that have this effect. In fact, the sulfur-containing amino acid methionine seems to help prevent the negative health effects of 1,2-dichloropropane and 1,2-dichloroethane.

Vitamin E has proven useful in lessening the toxic effects of very large doses of silver and preventing tricresyl phosphate poisoning. Vitamin B_{12} and nicotinic acid seem to protect the liver from damage done by carbon tetrachloride, and the B vitamin pyridoxine has been used by physicians to treat the toxic effects of carbon disulfide. The mineral selenium has proved quite useful in protecting the blood-forming organs from benzene, and vitamins A and C may be able to protect the ears from loud noises and help in repairing the damage that prolonged exposure to noise can cause.

It is important to remember that though these findings are encouraging, most are the results of work with animal models only, making it difficult to conclude with a high degree of certainty that the results will apply to humans. And, if they do apply, it is difficult to determine the quantities of particular nutrients needed to offer a worker protection against specific chemicals. For the moment, the best rule of thumb is to eat a diet that supplies at least the recommended dietary requirement of all nutrients.

Because of the potential importance of nutrition to workers in a variety of industries, we believe that nutrition education should become commonplace in large industries. Because much of the evidence cited in this chapter has yet to be carefully verified with controlled human studies, we do not believe there is sufficient justification to recommend that industries in which workers are exposed to chemical hazards provide their employees with nutritional supplements to help lower their risk of occupationally related disease. However, that does not mean that nutritional supplements will not offer workers some protection from the chemicals they work with, and many workers, given adequate education, may choose to take supplements on their own.

CHAPTER 8

Getting Well and Staying Healthy: How Drugs Affect Nutrition

Medications are a unique group of environmental chemicals. Unlike pollutants, which injure the body, drugs are deliberately taken to heal the body and cure disease. We welcome them because they bring relief or because they help us lead normal, healthy lives. But many drugs have side effects—some minor, some serious—which we grudgingly accept to derive the benefits of the medications. One type of side effect, though, need not occur at all.

When taken as prescribed, many medications cause nutritional deficiencies. Oral contraceptives, for example, increase the daily requirement for vitamin C and several B vitamins. Laxatives can shortchange the body of several important nutrients. On the other hand, some drugs may actually decrease one's need for nutrients and still others have side effects that can be alleviated with nutrition. This chapter describes some of those drug-nutrient interactions.

Nutritional deficiencies induced by drugs can leave the body vulnerable to the deleterious effects of various toxins and carcinogens, as noted elsewhere in this book. In this chapter, we will point out a few of these and direct you to the chapters where they are described in more detail.

THE PERILS OF THE PILL

When the first hormonal contraceptive pills were introduced in the 1950s, they were hailed as the perfect birth-control method. Nearly 100-percent effective when properly employed, they were easy to use and had fully reversible effects on the female reproductive system. In the nearly 30 years that the pill has been available, a number of side effects have come to light. Despite these disadvantages, oral contraceptives remain one of the most widely used methods of contraception in the United States.

Birth-control pills contain synthetic analogs of natural reproductive hormones. These manmade hormones interfere with the processes of ovulation, fertilization and implantation of fertilized eggs in the uterine lining. The most commonly used oral contraceptives are the combination pills that contain substances that behave like natural estrogens and progesterones, the hormones that regulate the female reproductive cycle.

Oral contraceptives do what they are designed to do quite well. But the same hormones that prevent pregnancy also cause such side effects as blood clots in the veins (especially in women over 35 who smoke), nausea, headaches, elevated blood pressure, vaginal discharges and depression, among other things. Use of the pill has also been linked to an increased risk of heart attacks, especially in women who smoke. On the other hand, research in the last few years suggests that women who use the pill are less likely to get uterine cancer and about half as likely as women who do not use the pill to get cancer of the ovaries.

In a small but not insignificant number of women, birth-control pills cause vitamin deficiencies. Several studies have found that users of oral contraceptives may suffer partial deficiencies of vitamins B_{12}, riboflavin, folic acid and, most importantly, B_6.

The effects of a B_6 deficiency may be manifested as depression, and in fact as many as one in four women taking the pill frequently suffer from irritability and depression, with the symptoms becoming more pronounced the longer the use of oral contraceptives continues. How reproductive hormones cause a nutritional deficiency that in turn triggers depression has become clearer over the last 20 years. The estrogen in the pill seems to speed the conversion by the body of tryptophan, an essential amino acid, to its more useful forms. Several of the enzymes involved in this process contain vitamin B_6. As the metabolism of tryptophan is increased by estrogen, greater enzyme activity occurs and more and more B_6 is used up.

Vitamin B_6 is also required to make a chemical known as 5-hydroxytryptamine, which seems to prevent depression. Studies of depressive illness have shown that a common denominator among sufferers of serious depression is an unusually low blood level of this compound. As more B_6 is used converting tryptophan, less and less is available to manufacture 5-hydroxytryptamine. Consequently, the concentration of this substance drops and depression sets in.

For pill users who suffer from depression, relief may be as simple as taking vitamin B supplements. Several studies have shown marked improvement and even total remission in depressed women treated in this manner. One team of scientists has recommended that all pill users take regular supplements of B_6, though this view is not shared by everyone working in the field.

Some researchers have argued that putting more B_6 into the bloodstream only steps up the transformation of tryptophan, doing little to overcome the B_6 shortage and creating a tryptophan deficiency in the process. Others have noted that compounds created when tryptophan is chemically transformed can cause cancer and diabetes in animals when present in larger-than-normal amounts. No one, however, has proposed that they pose a danger to humans.

Oral contraceptives can also deplete the body's supply of folic acid, another B vitamin. Although a small deficit of folic acid will not affect normal, healthy women, it may be a serious problem for a developing fetus. Folic acid is required for normal cell division, and in fact research has shown that a folic acid deficiency can cause birth defects in animals. Whether a minor folic acid deficiency induced by birth-control pills can harm a human fetus is a matter of controversy. However, it would seem wise for women who became pregnant shortly after discontinuing use of the pill, and in fact any woman carrying a child, to eat a diet rich in B vitamins. Chapter 3 lists some good dietary sources.

Vitamin A should also be on the minds of women who become pregnant shortly after going off the pill, but for a different reason. In 1971, Isabel Gal and her associates at Queen Charlotte's Maternity Hospital in London noticed that women on combination pills often have elevated plasma levels of vitamin A during certain portions of their menstrual cycles. The results were obtained with healthy women between the ages of 20 and 22, all of whom presumably ate a fairly normal diet. Gal also discovered that quantities of carotene, the precursor of vitamin A found in plants, dropped whenever vitamin A levels rose, suggesting that something was stimulating the conversion of carotene to vitamin A in the blood.

Several additional studies by Gal and by others confirmed the occurrence of a common, albeit minor, surplus of vitamin A in the blood of pill users. Gal hypothesized that estrogen steps up the production of a protein that binds with vitamin A in the bloodstream. An abundance of this protein may pull vitamin A out of storage and into the blood.

The levels of vitamin A in women who take the pill are far too low to be toxic and may, by promoting the normal growth of a class of tissue known as epithelium, prevent cancers in such organs as the uterus and ovaries. On the other hand, the results of animal studies have suggested that too much vitamin A circulating through the blood of a fetus can cause birth defects, just as too little folic acid can cause abnormal development. Only weak, circumstantial evidence exists to suggest that human fetuses suffer from elevated vitamin A levels, though.

In fact, one researcher has pointed out that the amount of vitamin A in the blood of pill users is no higher than the quantity normally found in the blood of pregnant women who take vitamin supplements, apparently without ill effects to the fetus. However, Gal has found that blood vitamin A levels normally drop dramatically in the first 12 weeks of pregnancy, perhaps to protect the fetus during the early stages of development when cell division is taking place at a very rapid rate. Gal has urged women to wait at least three months after ceasing use of the pill before conceiving, since it takes about that long for plasma vitamin A levels to return to normal. She also advised against the use of vitamin A supplements during pregnancy.

Oral contraceptives lower the concentration of vitamin C in the liver, adrenal glands and uterus of test animals. The pill seems to have the same effect on people, but the human studies done to date have all had important flaws. For instance, they failed to consider factors besides the pill that can deplete the body's vitamin C, such as aspirin, smoking and toxic chemicals. Although the findings are far from conclusive, the fact that a vitamin C deficiency can increase the body's susceptibility to a variety of toxins and carcinogens—including lead, ozone, pesticides and PCBs—suggests that it is best for pill users to eat a diet rich in vitamin C.

Oral contraceptives increase the absorption of calcium through the digestive tract. While extra calcium by itself usually poses little or no health risk, substances that aid calcium absorption also increase the uptake of heavy metals such as lead and cadmium. In fact, there is evidence that pill users often have elevated levels of copper, a metal that can be toxic in fairly small amounts, in their bodies.

Oral contraceptive users also tend to have an excess of vitamin K in their blood along with several proteins involved in blood clotting. It is possible that this excess vitamin K, which is required for normal clotting, may be the cause of two rare side effects of the pill, thrombophlebitis (blood clots in the veins) and thromboembolism (blood clots that travel to the lungs).

Because vitamin K is produced by bacteria in the intestine it would probably be difficult, if not impossible, to control one's intake of this nutrient. However, one can easily adjust one's intake of the B vitamins, and the evidence described in this chapter suggests that many women on the pill may need to consume extra B vitamins. In particular, the pill is capable of causing deficiencies of B_{12}, riboflavin, folic acid and B_6. A deficiency of B_6 may explain the symptoms of depression that plague a small number of women who take oral contraceptives. Unfortunately, scientists disagree about the best way to relieve the depression. Some have advocated supplements of B_6, while others have suggested that these supplements may actually aggravate the depression. We believe that the Food and Drug Administration, which regulates both vitamins and oral contraceptives, should address this issue and provide some guidance to women on the pill.

Women who become pregnant after discontinuing the use of the pill should carefully control their intake of two vitamins: vitamin A and folic acid. Pill users often suffer from a folic acid deficiency while having elevated levels of vitamin A. Both conditions have been associated with birth defects in animals, though no evidence exists that either can cause birth defects in people. However, to be on the safe side, women who conceive within three months after discontinuing pill use should consume rich sources of folic acid and avoid excessive consumption of vitamin A (providing that their diet is at least meeting the recommended dietary requirements).

The research we have examined also suggests that women on

oral contraceptives may need more vitamin C and less calcium than the average adult woman. However, this research is far from conclusive.

ASPIRIN AND VITAMIN C

Aspirin is the most commonly used pain killer in the United States. Taken alone or as part of dozens of cold remedies, headache pills, premenstrual tension relievers and medications for the treatment of arthritis, toothache and fever, aspirin is consumed by millions of people every day.

Known by its pharmacological name of acetylsalicylic acid, aspirin is not only an analgesic (pain reliever), but also one of the most effective treatments for fever and inflammation. It is not, of course, a perfect drug, since it has its share of side effects. A small number of people are allergic to aspirin and many others find that it irritates their stomachs. Aspirin also causes stomach bleeding, which in certain cases can be quite severe. And aspirin retards the normal clotting of blood.

These are not the only side effects of America's most popular medication. In the 1970s, confirming the results of research conducted 30 years earlier, aspirin was found to lower the concentration of vitamin C in certain types of blood cells. An aspirin dose of 600 milligrams (just under the amount in two typical tablets, the recommended adult dose) prevented blood cells from assimilating vitamin C. In theory, this could lower the ability of white blood cells to help fight off infections and destroy foreign matter and may account for aspirin's effects on blood clotting. Even when aspirin was taken with a large dose of vitamin C, much of the vitamin was lost in the urine and none was taken up by blood cells. Other research indicated that aspirin can rob many body tissues, not just blood cells, of vitamin C.

How aspirin affects the body's vitamin C stores seems to depend on whether the body is healthy or under the influence of a cold. Dr. C. W. M. Wilson in 1975 took white blood cells from subjects with colds and mixed them in suspension with aspirin and vitamin C. Rather than inhibit the absorption of the vitamin by the cells, the aspirin actually seemed to enhance it. This effect disappeared as the patients who donated the cells recovered from their colds. Whether this phenomenon accounts for any of vitamin C's supposed cold-fighting abilities is not known.

An occasional dose of aspirin to cure a headache or to bring down a fever will probably not threaten one's stores of vitamin C. This is a water-soluble vitamin, which means it is not retained by the body and must be replenished every day, whether aspirin is taken or not. But many people must take aspirin several times a day, every day of their lives. Among them are sufferers of rheumatoid arthritis, which causes painful inflammation and degeneration of the joints.

The pain of arthritis is often treated with large doses of aspirin, a less expensive and often equally effective alternative to other anti-inflammatory drugs such as cortisone and steroids. In the future, doctors may prescribe aspirin for other disorders. Recent and very preliminary findings suggest that small, daily doses of aspirin may lower the risk of heart attack, retard the development of cataracts in the elderly and, possibly, prove a useful treatment for cancer.

In a study of arthritis patients who take 12 or more 325-milligram aspirin tablets each day, the subjects were found to have abnormally low tissue levels of vitamin C. Since a deficiency of vitamin C can greatly increase stomach bleeding in those who take aspirin frequently, it is believed that arthritis patients who use aspirin also probably suffer from iron deficiencies. In fact, a number of researchers consider the chronic use of aspirin to be a leading cause of iron deficiency anemia in the United States.

In addition to its effects on vitamin C, aspirin has also been implicated as a cause of B vitamin deficiencies in heavy users. In one study, 71 percent of a group of 51 rheumatoid arthritis patients tested had below-normal tissue levels of folic acid. Aspirin and similar drugs may prevent folic acid from linking with a protein that normally carries it through the bloodstream, making it more likely to be removed from the blood by the kidneys.

It is unlikely that the normal use of aspirin will cause more than a temporary disruption of nutrition. However, long-term, heavy use of this medication can cause deficiencies of vitamin C and folic acid that can place the user at higher risk to a variety of environmental agents. For this reason, arthritis patients who use aspirin and any other heavy users should take a multivitamin or at least daily vitamin C and B complex supplements.

TREATING EPILEPSY AND DEPLETING VITAMINS

One to two million Americans, mostly children, suffer from epilepsy. It is estimated that anywhere from four to six percent of all children have at least one episode of convulsive seizures before reaching adulthood. The causes of seizure disorders include oxygen deprivation or injury during birth, congenital defects, genetic disorders, accidents, child abuse, brain tumors and drug abuse or withdrawal. While many sufferers endure the more serious grand mal seizures, which are characterized by loss of consciousness and violent muscle spasms, there are several other less serious forms of epilepsy in which the seizures are marked by such symptoms as momentary loss of consciousness, twitching limbs, aching stomach, occasional headaches, fluttering eyes, momentary loss of muscle tone and incoherent behavior.

The most serious forms of epilepsy can be treated with a class of drugs known as anticonvulsants. The *Physicians' Desk Reference,* a compendium of information about prescription medications, lists 17 types of anticonvulsants. Among those commonly prescribed are phenobarbital, butabarbital, pentobarbital—barbiturates also used as sedatives—diphenylhydantoin, primidone and phenytoin. All of these drugs have side effects, which range from nausea and headaches to loss of muscle coordination. Two of the more serious side effects have been linked to nutritional deficiencies caused by the drugs.

For many years physicians have observed anemia and other signs of inadequate red blood cell production in patients taking anticonvulsant drugs. Most researchers agree that the blood disorders are caused by a deficiency of folic acid. The drugs apparently reduce the absorption of folic acid and speed its removal into the urine.

Severe deficiencies of folic acid can cause changes in behavior as well as respiratory tract, heart and digestive disorders and severe anemia. The blood and behavioral disorders can be relieved with large doses of folic acid. However, in some cases, the cure can be as damaging as the disease. Several researchers have found that the administration of large doses of folic acid can trigger seizures in animals. In fact, when injected into the brain cavity of healthy rats and dogs, folic acid sets off convulsions.

Why folic acid causes convulsions is not clear, though there have been no known cases of vitamin-induced seizures in people. Anticonvulsants may prevent the conversion of folic acid to a compound that is capable of crossing the barrier from the blood to the central nervous system where it causes seizures. It has also been theorized that large doses of folic acid may deplete the anticonvulsants circulating through the bloodstream of an epileptic patient, making the patient more susceptible to stimuli that can trigger seizures.

Large doses of folic acid can also cause a minor deficiency of vitamin B_{12}. However, unless an epileptic already suffers from a marginal B_{12} deficiency, this effect is usually of little concern.

Another serious problem seen in epileptics who take anticonvulsants is bone softening. Although rare in the general population, rickets (in children) and osteomalacia (in adults) are seen in a significant percentage of chronic users of anticonvulsant drugs. In fact, diagnostic x-rays in a number of studies have detected bone changes in anywhere from 15 to 80 percent of patients studied.

When a child gets rickets, his or her bones fail to mineralize and instead stay soft. The weight of a child's body causes the legs to bow. The head, chest and pelvis can also become deformed. In adolescents and adults osteomalacia affects fully developed bones, causing a loss of minerals, which leads to softness and malformation. Rickets and osteomalacia are caused by a deficiency of vitamin D. In fact, both conditions respond to treatment with vitamin D, especially a form known as 25-hydroxycholecalciferol. It is thought that anticonvulsants enhance the activity of enzymes in the liver that attack foreign chemicals and drugs. Vitamin D is probably an innocent victim of these enzymes.

It is apparent from this research that patients who take anticonvulsant drugs are at high risk to developing a vitamin D deficiency great enough to impair normal development and maintenance of bones. For this reason, these patients should be extremely careful to eat a good source of vitamin D every day. As noted in Chapter 3, fish, fish oils, fortified milk, butter and egg yolks all contain vitamin D. Since a few of these sources are also high in fat or cholesterol, a daily vitamin D supplement may be a better way to ensure an adequate intake of this vitamin.

LAXATIVES AND MALNUTRITION

Old wives' tales die hard. Many Americans still chart their physical well-being by the regularity of their bowel movements. If they do not defecate every day they assume something is out of balance and try to compensate. Nearly $300 million is spent each year on the most common form of compensation: laxatives.

Laxatives, or cathartics as physicians and pharmacists call them, act in a variety of ways. Stimulants contain chemicals, such as phenolphthalein or castor oil, that induce bowel muscles to contract and speed the passage of the waste material. Lubricants soften the stool. Wetting agents moisten the feces and salines draw water into the bowel to ease the movement of the waste. Bulk formers, the so-called natural laxatives, expand and soften the stool.

Despite what multi-million-dollar advertising campaigns suggest, laxatives are rarely needed, except when prescribed by a physician. But, caught up in the myth of daily defecation, millions of Americans dose themselves repeatedly with pleasant-tasting liquids and convenient pills and suppositories. In doing so, they risk all-too-common side effects of laxative overuse—cramps, diarrhea, dehydration and weakened intestinal muscles.

An important class of laxative abusers are a group consisting mostly of young women who are torn between a compulsion to eat and a desire to be thin. While many literally starve their bodies, others repeatedly overeat and then purge themselves of the food they have just eaten. Some choose vomiting for the purging stage of their mental illness, but many others rely on overdoses of laxatives. This binge-purge syndrome, known as bulimia or bulimiarexia, is becoming a major public health problem.

The majority of abusers of laxatives, however, seek only to

maintain their physical or mental well-being. But as they purge their digestive tracts, they rob their bodies of vitamins and minerals. Frequent use of mineral oil, a once-popular lubricant-type laxative, can easily cause deficiencies of vitamins A, D and K. Cases of rickets and osteomalacia (adult bone softening) have also been documented in mineral oil users.

Because they are potent and fast-acting, the stimulants are the most commonly used and abused laxatives. Using these medications too often can bring on malnutrition, since laxatives not only prevent the body from absorbing enough vitamin C and vitamin D, but also prevent the assimilation of adequate quantities of protein. Stimulants probably act by causing intestinal hurry, a quickening of the bowel muscles that speeds the waste through the digestive tract before the nutritional contents of the food can be adequately transferred to the bloodstream. So, though heavy laxative users may eat adequate diets, they can still suffer from nutritional deficiencies.

Vitamin deficiencies may increase the laxative user's susceptibility to many toxins and carcinogens. Many of these are described elsewhere in this book. Some of the more important are nitrites, mercury, pesticides and PCBs (Chapter 5); hydrocarbon carcinogens and alcohol (Chapter 9); lead, cadmium and ozone (Chapter 6); and many industrial chemicals (Chapter 7).

The best way to prevent vitamin deficiencies brought on by the overuse of laxatives is to simply stop using laxatives, or to at least limit their use to times when they are absolutely necessary. Unless the bowel movements have become extremely irregular or you are suffering from other lower digestive tract symptoms such as chronic constipation or bleeding, there is probably no need to worry about so-called irregularity. If you are concerned about the condition of your bowel, a trip to the doctor is in order, not a trip to the medicine cabinet for a dose of laxative. But, if you must take laxatives on a regular basis, you should also consider taking a multivitamin supplement every day.

ANTACIDS AND SOFT BONES

When Americans are not trying to overcome irregularity, they are probably fighting off indigestion. The overuse of antacids, such as aluminum hydroxide, can also cause nutrient depletion. Antacids combine with phosphates in the digestive tract, sweetening sour stomachs and also blocking the absorption of phosphorus, a mineral that makes up part of the structure of bones.

Occasional use of antacids probably does no harm. It is when these medications are taken routinely that problems arise. In one case related by Daphne Roe, an authority on drug-induced nutritional deficiencies, a 49-year-old woman took antacids containing aluminum hydroxide regularly for months to alleviate severe heartburn caused by a hiatus hernia. When she finally visited a physician, she was suffering from pain in her bones, weakness and difficulty in walking. Upon examination, she showed signs of osteomalacia, which her physican attributed to her overuse of antacids.

As with laxatives, the best way to avoid antacid-induced nutritional deficiency is to avoid the overuse of antacids. Frequent or prolonged heartburn or indigestion can be signs of an ulcer or a heart attack. It is best to consult with a physician rather than using antacids to cope with these symptoms. If, on the advice of a physician, you are taking antacids on a regular basis, you should also discuss whether you need a regular phosphorus supplement.

ANTIBIOTICS: PROBLEMS WITH THE MIRACLE DRUGS

Antibiotics have been rightfully hailed as wonder drugs. Acting quickly and effectively to destroy disease-causing bacteria, they have revolutionized medical practice and reduced the death rate from bacterial infections. Unfortunately, many antibiotics impede the absorption of nutrients from the digestive tract. With most antibiotic drugs this minor side effect is outweighed by the benefits of the medication. However, one class of bacterial fighters can cause serious deficiencies.

Broad-spectrum antibiotics like neomycin, which are effective against a wide variety of microorganisms, have been known to produce temporary malnutrition. In most cases, the symptoms are short-lived and disappear soon after the use of the drug is discontinued. Many researchers believe antibiotics alter the shape of the villi (the tiny projections from the lining of the small intestine through which nutrients are absorbed) and consequently interfere with their normal functioning. The nutrients most commonly affected are sodium, potassium, calcium, vitamin B_{12}, iron, fats and certain amino acids. Neomycin is also known to destroy the bacteria that populate the lower digestive tract and that also manufacture vitamin K and the B vitamins biotin and thiamine (B_1), so deficiencies of these nutrients are also possible in neomycin users.

Tetracycline, another broad-spectrum antibiotic, is capable of causing kidney damage, though research with rats and dogs has shown that large doses of vitamin C can prevent this side effect. The vitamin apparently enhances the excretion of the drug by the kidneys and lowers its concentration in the bloodstream.

Most people will use broad-spectrum antibiotics rarely if at all, so the disruption of normal nutrition will not cause serious problems. However, because these drugs are known to lower the digestive tract absorption of several nutrients, good nutrition is all the more important during antibiotic therapy.

LAETRILE AND VITAMIN C: A HAZARDOUS COMBINATION

After much discussion and testing and many clinical trials, one conclusion can be made about laetrile, the supposed anticancer drug made from apricot pits. It does not appear to work. But, despite the lack of evidence to support claims about laetrile, many cancer patients continue to turn to it.

One active ingredient in laetrile is thought to be cyanide, a highly poisonous substance. Cyanide is a fast-acting toxin that kills cells by preventing them from converting food into energy. Lower doses can cause headaches, weakness, disorientation and nausea. Large amounts of vitamin C are thought to increase the toxicity of cyanide by using up chemicals that are essential to the breakdown and deactivation of cyanide by the body.

A few researchers, most notably Nobel laureate Linus Pauling, have advocated the use of megadoses of vitamin C to fight cancer. It is not surprising, therefore, that many patients who try laetrile also take massive amounts of this vitamin. This combination probably does no good at all and may, in fact, be hazardous. Even if laetrile is taken alone, vitamin C intake should be closely monitored along with the toxic effects of the cyanide in laetrile.

OTHER DRUG/NUTRIENT INTERACTIONS

Antihistamines

Found in many cold remedies, hay fever and allergy medications and sleep aids, antihistamines interfere with the activity of histamine, an irritant released by specialized cells in the presence of foreign matter, pollen, viruses and other potential allergens. Antihistamines can enhance the excretion of vitamin C, depleting this water-soluble vitamin.

Colchicine

Used to treat gout, this drug can cause deficiencies of vitamin B_{12}, sodium, potassium and fats.

Diuretics

Prescribed for high blood pressure and other conditions that call for removal of body fluids, some diuretics can cause magnesium, zinc and potassium deficiencies.

Chelating Agents

These are used to treat poisoning by lead and other heavy metals. They latch on to and remove the metals from the body. They can also cause a deficiency of zinc, an essential mineral.

Drugs into Carcinogens

A number of medications belong to a class of organic chemicals known as amines. When mixed in the stomach with an adequate amount of another chemical, nitrite, the drugs can react to form nitrosamines, potent carcinogens. This is the same chemical reaction that occurs when nitrites in cured meat react with the amines in other foods (see Chapter 5).

Drugs that may enter into such reactions include tetracycline, a broad-spectrum antibiotic; piperazine, a drug for treating infections by roundworm or pinworm; phenmetrazine hydrochloride, a short-term weight-loss aid for the treatment of obesity; ethambutol, a potent diuretic; and disulfiram, which causes an unpleasant reaction when one drinks alcohol and is therefore used in the treatment of alcoholism.

Vitamin C can prevent the chemical reaction that occurs between nitrites and amines when it is taken along with these drugs. A few scientists have recommended that all drugs that contain amines be formulated with vitamin C, and in fact a few, such as certain forms of tetracycline, already are.

CONCLUSION: THE UNMENTIONED SIDE EFFECTS OF DRUGS

Despite their potential seriousness, drug-induced nutritional deficiencies are rarely mentioned to patients who receive prescription or nonprescription drugs. Unfortunately, physicians are often not aware that the drugs they prescribe can affect their patient's nutrition. This ignorance is not always the fault of the doctors, since medical textbooks and references on medications often fail to address the nutritional side effects of medications.

It is safe to say that many medications available today have some effect on nutrition. Some cause nutritional deficiencies. Oral contraceptives can cause deficiencies of vitamin C and several B vitamins. Aspirin can cause a deficiency of vitamin C in a healthy body. Anticonvulsants can cause serious shortages of vitamin D. Laxatives, antacids and broad-spectrum antibiotics can cause deficiencies of several vitamins and minerals.

Oral contraceptives can actually diminish the body's requirement for vitamins A and K and the mineral calcium. In fact, excess vitamin K created by the pill may be responsible for the blood clots that appear in the veins of a small number of women on the pill. The effectiveness of some medications is diminished by excesses of nutrients. Vitamin K can interfere with the action of anticoagulant drugs and calcium can impair the performance of tetracycline and similar antibiotics.

Since your physician and pharmacist may not be aware of many of these interactions, you will, unfortunately, be on your own in dealing with the nutritional effects of medications. The examples cited in this chapter are only some of the many drugs that seem to affect the body's requirements for nutrients. For the drugs we did not deal with, a general rule of thumb is that most medications that do affect nutrition seem to cause deficiencies of one or more nutrients. So a balanced diet is a must when taking medications.

CHAPTER 9

Playing with Fire: How Our Lifestyles Affect Our Susceptibility to Pollutants

Air and water pollution, food contaminants, industrial chemicals and prescription drugs are types of chemicals we often cannot avoid. In fact, we often accept them as necessary evils—unfortunate but inescapable facts of life. But while we grudgingly reconcile ourselves to this chemical fate, we sometimes willingly expose ourselves to toxins and carcinogens that may pose a greater risk to our health than the chemical sea around us.

The habits, idiosyncrasies and other behaviors that collectively make up our lifestyle can markedly affect our propensity to disease and the length and quality of our lives. Deciding to drive a car, for example, means taking a serious risk, since more people die each year in traffic accidents than from most life-threatening diseases. Likewise, choosing to live in a poorly ventilated brick house, where the radioactive compounds normally present in bricks may create dangerous levels of radioactive radon gas, involves an element of risk, since it can increase the odds that we will get cancer. This chapter will focus on three behaviors, three choices we make that can have significant impacts on our health: smoking, drinking alcohol and our diet.

Inhaling the smoke from a burning cigarette brings the smoker into intimate contact with a mixture of poisons and cancer-causing chemicals. By repeating this contact several times a day, day after day, the smoker provides more-than-ample opportunity for the smoke to cause tissue damage and, worse, to initiate cancer. Little

163

wonder that the smoking of cigarettes (and pipes, cigars and marijuana cigarettes) is one of the most serious public health problems in this country.

A somewhat less frequent, though no less serious, problem is that posed by heavy drinking. It is estimated that ten million Americans are problem drinkers, consuming alcohol to excess on a regular basis. In addition to the emotional damage alcoholism inflicts on the sufferer and others in his life, heavy drinking has a physical price tag as well. Alcohol has the ability to damage many organs in the body, but two, the brain and the liver, take the brunt of the injury. Cirrhosis of the liver, cancer and behavioral disorders are too often the consequences of a lifetime of drinking.

Diet is the third aspect of our lifestyles we will deal with in this chapter. Several components of our diet seem to markedly affect our chances of developing cancers. For example, fiber, the parts of plants that we cannot digest, may help prevent cancers of the colon, while fats in excess may promote colon cancer as well as cancers of the breast and other tissues.

We will conclude the chapter with a look at a lifestyle that may be worth emulating. Members of the Seventh-Day Adventist faith do not, by and large, smoke or drink, and they eat a diet low in fats and rich in fiber. As a group, they display a lower incidence of cancer, heart disorders and other serious diseases than the rest of us and they tend to live longer. They are living proof that the way we live our lives can determine to a significant extent how long we may live and how healthy we may be.

SMOKING: A BREATH OF DEADLY AIR

There is a product widely manufactured in the United States that probably contributes to the deaths of over 200,000 people each year. It routinely exposes anyone who uses it, and anyone nearby, to a gaseous blend of carcinogens, heavy metals and other toxic compounds. Those who employ this product on a regular basis have been found to have twice the normal levels of radioactive lead and polonium in their rib bones and lung tissue.

The health hazards associated with the use of this product have been recognized for many years, but its manufacture has been allowed to continue unabated and virtually unregulated. A federal panel concluded in 1982 that this product is unquestionably linked with a constantly growing incidence in the United States of cancer of the lungs and other organs. It is now believed that as many as 75 percent of all lung cancers in this country are primarily due to use of this commodity.

Surprisingly, while the weight of evidence against this product grows each year, to date the strongest action taken by the federal government to control its use has been a regulation requiring a small label warning users that the product is dangerous to their health. Not only has the federal government failed to control or prohibit the manufacture of this product, but it also spends millions of dollars each year to subsidize production of the raw material needed to make it.

The product, of course, is the cigarette. Spurred by billions of dollars of high-powered advertising and undeterred by national antismoking campaigns by such groups as the American Lung Association, millions of Americans smoke cigarettes. Once primarily a habit of men, cigarette smoking has gained an impressive female following. As a result, lung cancer rates for women are beginning to rise (Figure 4). Emulating parents and peers, teenagers by the millions continue to take up the habit each year, assuring that the health effects of cigarettes will be with us for many years to come.

The effects of smoking are many and have been well documented. They range from an increased propensity to colds to an elevated risk of several types of cancer. In between are a higher risk of emphysema, a debilitating disease of the lungs, and a higher-than-normal incidence of heart disease and arteriosclerosis. Among the cancers smoking has been linked to are carcinomas of the nasal sinuses, throat, pharynx, larynx, kidney, bladder, pancreas and lungs.

As Figure 4 shows, there can be little doubt that smoking and lung cancer are strongly linked. As the consumption of cigarettes by Americans has climbed each year, the rate of lung cancer has risen in step. In addition, studies on the relationship between the number of cigarettes smoked by an individual and the resulting risk of lung cancer show a clear, straight-line relationship.

The health problems associated with cigarette smoking (and cigar, pipe and marijuana smoking, for that matter) are not at all

Figure 4
Relationship Between Cigarette Smoking and Lung Cancer

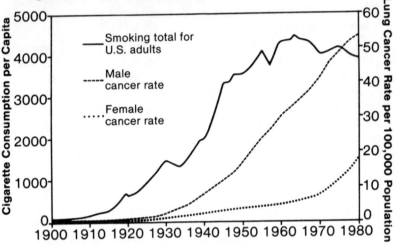

As this graph shows, cigarette smoking and lung cancer are unquestionably associated. The rate of lung cancer among American adults has risen in step with the increasing consumption of cigarettes in this country. However, as you can see, there is a long latency period between the increase in cigarette smoking and the rise in the lung-cancer rate. American men became heavy smokers long before American women, and as a result, the lung-cancer rate for women has begun to skyrocket only within the last few decades. (Cigarette-consumption figures from the United States Department of Agriculture; cancer statistics from the National Cancer Institute.)

surprising once you realize just what is in tobacco smoke. As a look at Table 3 will show, the smoke from a burning cigarette contains a considerable number of toxic and carcinogenic substances. Cancer-causing hydrocarbons such as benzo(a)pyrene; toxic heavy metals like lead, cadmium and nickel; radioactive compounds like polonium-210 and lead-210; and an assortment of sticky tars and nicotine make up the foul-smelling conglomeration that enters the air from both ends of a cigarette.

A proposed State of Illinois environmental standard for the

TABLE 3 | SOME OF THE TOXIC AND CARCINOGENIC SUBSTANCES THAT HAVE BEEN FOUND IN CIGARETTE SMOKE

Toxins

Acetaldehyde	Nicotine
Acetone	Nitrogen dioxide
Acetonitrile	Particulate matter
Ammonia	Phenol
Argon	Pyridine
Butylamine	Other gases
Cadmium	
Carbon dioxide	**Carcinogens and**
Carbon monoxide	**Suspected Carcinogens**
Creosol	Benzene
Endrin	Chrysene
DDT	Formaldehyde
Hydrogen sulfide	Lead-210
Hydrogen cyanide	Polonium-210
Lead	Benzo(a)pyrene
Methane	Dibenzo(a,h)anthracene
Methyl alcohol	Dibenzo(a,h)pyrene
Nickel compounds	Other hydrocarbons

toxic metal cadmium would allow an accumulation of five milligrams in the body of an average person over the course of 45 years. Someone who smokes a pack of cigarettes a day will accumulate that much cadmium from the cigarettes alone in just 20 years. The smoke from one cigarette contains 200 to 800 parts per million of carbon monoxide, a gas that binds very strongly with hemoglobin in red blood cells, preventing those cells from carrying oxygen to the body's tissues. Smoking one pack a day can result in five to six percent of the hemoglobin in one's blood becoming bound up with carbon monoxide.

Nitrogen dioxide, an ingredient of urban air pollution, is also a component of smoke. Tobacco smoke can contain up to 300 parts per million of nitrogen dioxide, with the largest amounts found in cigar and pipe smoke. As a comparison, the United States EPA ambient air quality standard for nitrogen dioxide is 0.5 part per million. In the lungs, nitrogen dioxide can combine with water to form nitrous and nitric acids, highly irritating compounds that may be related to the onset of emphysema in smokers.

Noxious, toxic and carcinogenic chemicals are only part of the problem with cigarette smoke. The chemicals are components of a foul blend of substances that hinder the ability of the body to protect itself against chemicals and other foreign invaders. The smoke paralyzes cilia, tiny hairlike projections that line the air passages leading to the lungs. The cilia normally catch foreign matter and push it out of the air passages with rhythmic, wavelike movements. Cigarette smoke anesthetizes the cilia and causes the secretion of excess mucus in the airways. The mucus drowns the cilia and also traps particles of smoke next to the lining of the respiratory tract, increasing the odds that irritations, cellular damage or cancer will result.

Cadmium and Emphysema

After several years of heavy smoking, the constant irritation of the air passages may cause them to constrict, making breathing more difficult. In time, the lining of the passages may weaken and become inflamed, leaving the respiratory tract more susceptible to infection by microorganisms. Eventually, the tissues of the lungs themselves begin to lose their elasticity and the tiny air sacs where oxygen passes into the bloodstream expand and contract with greater and greater difficulty. If heavy smoking continues, the lining of the lungs can deteriorate further, sometimes resulting in a debilitating disease known as emphysema.

In emphysema, the air sacs remain filled with air at all times, whereas normal air sacs contract during exhalation to expel stale air. Because the air sacs do not contract properly, the movement of air into and out of the lungs is diminished, as is the movement of oxygen into the bloodstream. As the disease progresses, even mild exercise may leave the victim breathless.

Work by Dr. Parimal Chowdhury and colleagues at the University of Arkansas for Medical Sciences and the New Jersey Medical School now suggests that the heavy metal cadmium may be a cause of smoking-induced emphysema. The initial clue to this discovery was the fact that industrial workers who handle cadmium and breathe in cadmium fumes have an unusually high rate of emphysema. Added to this was the finding that, in experiments with animals, emphysema can be induced by lowering the ability of the body to inhibit the activity of an enzyme called serum-alpha-1-antitrypsin.

The function of antitrypsin is to inactivate another enzyme known as trypsin. Trypsin is best known as a digestive enzyme that breaks down protein in the small intestine. But it is also produced by cells known as macrophages, which surround and digest bacteria and particles of foreign matter in the body. When the tissues of the lungs are damaged by cigarette smoke, macrophages congregate in the tissue and attempt to digest the particles and tars of the smoke. In the process, some of the macrophages are destroyed. They break open, spilling their contents, including trypsin, among the lung cells. Under normal conditions, serum-alpha-1-antitrypsin keeps the spilled trypsin in check. However, if there is not enough antitrypsin in the blood serum, the trypsin may begin to break down proteins in the membranes of the lung cells, just as it acts on proteins in the digestive tract. The researchers found that cadmium seems to produce emphysema not by acting directly on lung tissue but by causing a deficiency of serum-alpha-1-antitrypsin.

Chowdhury and his colleagues also noted that the effects of cadmium on antitrypsin are short-lived. In fact, 24 hours after a single exposure to cadmium, the level of the enzyme was back to normal. This implies that smokers can cut their chances of developing emphysema simply by kicking the habit, providing the disease has not progressed too far. The proper diet may also offer smokers some protection against cadmium. For more on the effect of the diet on cadmium, see Chapter 6.

Cyanide and Amblyopia

Among the many other components of cigarette smoke are molecules that contain the cyanide ion. A simple molecule consisting of a carbon atom bound to a nitrogen atom (CN), cyanide is an intensely poisonous substance. Hydrogen cyanide, one of the cyanides in cigarette smoke, inhibits the activity of certain enzymes, including those that are crucial for the effective production of energy in the body.

Analyses of the urine of smokers have confirmed that they are indeed exposed to abnormally high amounts of the cyanide ion. For example, the urine of smokers generally contains higher-than-normal levels of thiocyanate, a compound that results when cyanide is detoxified in the body. The fact that few smokers seem to suffer symptoms of cyanide poisoning attests to the ability of the body to deal with most of the cyanide in cigarette smoke. Vitamin B_{12} seems to be the front line of the body's defense.

Vitamin B_{12} exists in two forms: vitamins B_{12} and B_{12a}. In the 1950s, it was discovered that B_{12a} can bind tightly with cyanide, diminishing its effects on the body. The B_{12} form has had no effect on cyanide, at least in animal tests. In a normal body, B_{12a} is the more prevalent form of the vitamin. But since most of a smoker's B_{12a} is used up fighting off cyanide, the B_{12} form seems to predominate in smokers' blood.

When cyanide toxicity is expressed in smokers, it is generally seen as tobacco or toxic amblyopia, a dimming of vision. In 1954, researchers injected sufferers of toxic amblyopia with large doses of vitamin B_{12a} and were able to clear up the symptoms in all cases. In fact, later in the 1950s it was found that amblyopia sufferers have a general deficiency of vitamin B_{12} in both of its forms, and treatment with the vitamin has since become the standard cure.

Lung Cancer and Vitamin A

As mentioned earlier, smoking causes cancer in several organs, including the lungs, the bladder and the throat. All of these organs have one important characteristic in common: they are all partially made up of a type of tissue known as epithelium. Epithelium forms many of the body's boundary layers—the skin for example, as well as the lining of the lungs, urinary tract, circulatory system and other organs. Epithelium protects the body, helps it absorb food and allows it to secrete hormones and to make the reproductive cells—eggs and sperm—with which it creates new generations.

It has long been known that the normal growth and development of the epithelial tissue of numerous organs is dependent on vitamin A. What is just now becoming clear is that vitamin A may play a key role in preventing or reversing cancers of epithelium, such as those caused by smoking cigarettes. These chemopreventive and chemotherapeutic roles seem to be related to the ability of vitamin A to promote and maintain what is called differentiation in epithelial cells.

Differentiation is the process by which cells become specialized, performing specific functions in specific tissues in the body. The human body begins as a single cell that contains in its chromosomes the information to make a complete, functioning organism. This single cell then begins to divide, first forming a clump of cells that are all perfect copies of the original. As the individual develops, from clump to embryo to fetus to infant, cells take on highly specialized functions. Certain genes in each cell are somehow turned off and others, those related to the cell's function, are turned on.

Vitamin A not only seems to be essential to development, but also must be present to keep fully differentiated epithelial cells from reverting to their less specialized origins, a process known as dedifferentiation. This process, it is believed, precedes and signals the transformation of normal body cells into cancer cells. Interestingly, cancers in the organs dependent on vitamin A for normal differentiation account for over 60 percent of all cancer deaths.

The association between vitamin A and cell growth was known as early as 1926, when a Japanese scientist named Fujimaki noticed that papillomas, benign tumors of the skin and mucous membranes, formed in the stomachs of rats fed a vitamin-A-deficient diet. In the 1940s and 1950s, it was discovered that rats fed a diet deficient in vitamin A were also more likely to develop cancers when exposed to certain chemical carcinogens.

Knowing that a lack of vitamin A could increase the odds of epithelial cells' reverting to a precancerous state, scientists hypothesized that when administered in greater-than-required amounts, vitamin A might make epithelium less likely to dedifferentiate and therefore less susceptible to the effects of chemical carcinogens. In fact, it was believed, large amounts of vitamin A administered to an organism in which an epithelial cancer was already established might actually cause the tumor to shrink or disappear.

Support for this hypothesis was first obtained in the 1960s, when it was found that a large dose of vitamin A given to hamsters along with DMBA, a chemical carcinogen found in cigarette smoke, could lower the incidence of cancers of the cervix. Other work showed that vitamin A applied to the skin or fed to test animals could retard the progression of, and in some cases completely prevent, cancers of the esophagus, stomach and intestine in animals exposed to carcinogens, such as benzo(a)pyrene and DMBA.

Later work confirmed these early findings. A 1975 study found that vitamin A can reverse precancerous cell changes following exposure to certain cancer-causing agents in a cell culture. Michael Sporn, a leading cancer researcher with the National Cancer Institute, noted in 1976 that cancers of the epithelium in the bronchial tubes (one of the most common human cancers and one form of respiratory tract cancer linked conclusively with cigarette smoking) could be reversed with vitamin A treatment. The fact that many people whose diets are apparently meeting the United States RDA for vitamin A get these and other forms of epithelial cancer, he said, may indicate that the RDA is not adequate and should be reviewed in light of its ability as a cancer preventer.

Vitamin A has severe limitations as a cancer fighter for humans, though. When administered in doses high enough to reverse the course of cancer, it may be quite toxic and can cause liver damage. Also, it tends to accumulate in certain organs, especially the liver, and even at high doses may not reach cancer sites in adequate quantities. For these reasons, work over the past decade has focused on vitamin A mimics known as synthetic retinoids, and on beta-carotene, a precursor of vitamin A found in plants, which is apparently not toxic, even when consumed in high amounts in the diet.

Since 1974, it has been known that vitamin A mimics, which can be made in the laboratory, are both less toxic and offer more protection against tumors than natural vitamin A. These retinoids are produced by altering portions of the vitamin A molecule. Of the many possible variations, some are less toxic than natural vitamin A, making them suitable for administration in higher-than-normal doses. A number of these are also more effective in controlling dedifferentiation than natural vitamin A, giving them increased utility as cancer fighters. But the problem in cancer prevention and treatment is getting these chemotherapeutic or chemopreventive agents to the cancer site.

Work is underway to develop retinoids that will reach specific sites in the body in greater concentrations than can be achieved with natural vitamin A. One form already developed, called 13-*cis*-retinoic acid, has proved in animal tests to be effective in preventing cancers of the bladder and lungs. A trial involving the treatment of patients with bladder cancer has been underway since 1978. Tests of the effects of other vitamin A mimics on breast cancer patients are planned. Many tests such as these will be necessary to determine whether vitamin A analogs are the cancer fighters of the future.

But even as these studies are being performed, evidence has been gathered that indicates that the amount of vitamin A one consumes as beta-carotene may have a profound impact on one's chances of getting lung cancer. In the November 1981 issue of the British medical journal *Lancet,* Richard Shekelle and his colleagues at the Rush-Presbyterian-St. Luke's Medical Center in Chicago, the Harvard Medical School in Boston, the University of Michigan School of Nursing in Ann Arbor and the Northwestern University School of Medicine in Chicago reported that the intake of beta-carotene in the diets of more than 2,000 middle-aged men was inversely related to the incidence of lung cancer during the course of a long-term study.

The study began in 1957, when 2,107 male employees of a Western Electric Company plant in metropolitan Chicago were randomly selected and interviewed to determine the types of foods they normally ate. The participants were examined annually until 1969, and then again nine years after that. At the end of the study, the researchers determined how many of the men had contracted or died from cancer. They found that, as expected, the length of time the subjects had smoked was positively correlated with the onset of cancer. They also found that those who developed lung cancer tended to have below-normal levels of beta-carotene in their bloodstreams throughout the study. The amount of vitamin A they consumed as retinol, the type of vitamin A in animal tissues, did not seem to affect the development of lung cancer.

Unfortunately, Shekelle and his colleagues were not able to make precise estimates of the amount of vitamin A as carotene or retinol their subjects consumed. They relied on statistical estimates based on questionnaires filled out by the subjects. In addition, the authors expressed intake of the vitamins as retinol and carotene indexes, which are not directly translatable into standard units.

Therefore, it is difficult to say whether the subjects who got lung cancer did, in fact, consume the Recommended Dietary Allowance of vitamin A, or whether those who did not get cancer consumed excess vitamin A.

On the other hand, it is important to realize that the National Research Council's Recommended Dietary Allowances (RDAs) for the vitamin were designed to prevent night blindness, and do not yet take into consideration vitamin A's effect on normal cell differentiation. It is known that quantities of vitamin A above 100,000 international units (IUs) are generally toxic, but what of quantities between this extreme and the 5,000-IU RDA for an adult male? Some researchers have said that not only are diets with excess vitamin A (below grossly toxic levels) safe, but they are also, in fact, quite beneficial. Michael Sporn of the National Cancer Institute has asserted that people who eat only the RDA of vitamin A may not be sufficiently protected against environmental carcinogens. Several other researchers have made similar claims. It would seem imperative that the RDAs be critically assessed in light of this new information.

Smoking cigarettes is an obvious health hazard. The smoke from a burning cigarette contains a toxic and carcinogenic blend of chemicals. In addition to the substances we have covered in this section there is acetaldehyde (discussed in the following section on alcohol), lead and nitrogen dioxide (discussed in Chapter 6) and many others. While proper nutrition cannot serve as a total shield against the chemical hazards in cigarette smoke, it can at least offer some protection against several of the dangerous substances in smoke. Cadmium can cause a deficiency of an enzyme known as serum-alpha-1-antitrypsin, which may allow trypsin to digest the proteins in lung cells and cause emphysema. Zinc and vitamins C and E may reduce cadmium toxicity and slow its absorption into the body (as noted in Chapter 6). Cyanide in smoke can cause a blurring of the vision, a condition that can be cured with vitamin B_{12}. The activity of the many potent cancer-causing agents in cigarette smoke may be foiled by supplements of vitamin A, in particular, a form called carotene, which helps prevent cells from reverting to a more primitive stage of development, a first step in cancer. Table 4 lists some good sources of carotene.

But eating carrots to ward off lung cancer from smoking is not the best way to protect one's health. A much better solution, one

TABLE 4 | GOOD SOURCES OF CAROTENE

Food	Serving	Carotene (micrograms)
Collard greens	1 cup cooked	8,892
Spinach	1 cup cooked	8,748
Spinach	1 cup raw	2,676
Squashes:		
butternut	1 cup	7,872
hubbard	1 cup	5,904
acorn	1 cup	1,722
yellow	1 cup	636
zucchini	1 cup	5,544
Cantaloupes	½ fruit	5,544
Carrots	1 raw	4,758
Beet greens	1 cup cooked	4,440
Broccoli	1 cup cooked	2,320
Apricots	1 fruit	1,734
Papayas	1 cup	1,470
Prunes	1 cup	1,302
Peaches	1 large	1,218
Watermelon	1 cup	564

that will drastically lower one's risk of lung cancer and the many other ills caused by smoking, is simply to stop smoking.

ALCOHOL: ASSAULT ON THE LIVER

The liver may well be the most versatile organ in the human body. Weighing over four pounds in the average adult, it is certainly the largest human organ. In its four sections or lobes are cells that aid in blood clotting, help break down red blood cells when they are worn out, store food, make the digestive chemical bile and deactivate or activate drugs and harmful chemicals. Served by two separate blood supplies, the liver is a complex factory and chemical treatment plant all rolled into one.

While the liver is a fairly durable organ, it is susceptible to diseases brought on by a variety of environmental agents. One of the most common causes of liver disease is a strong nervous system depressant known as ethanol, ethyl alcohol or just plain alcohol. Repeated exposure to alcohol can destroy liver cells. If the damage is not too severe or the duration of exposure too long, the liver can repair itself. In the livers of those who drink heavily, though, damaged liver cells may be replaced with connective tissue instead of new liver cells. Connective tissue may infiltrate more and more of the liver until it is bloated and unable to perform its functions. This condition, known as cirrhosis, frequently ends in a painful death.

Cirrhosis is not the only health problem to which heavy drinkers are prone. Alcohol kills nerve cells in the brain, which may be one reason long-time alcoholics are subject to loss of memory, hallucinations and paranoia. Alcoholics (particularly those who already suffer from cirrhosis) also have an unusually high incidence of liver cancer and cancers of the mouth, pharynx, larynx and esophagus. In fact, esophageal cancer is seven times more common among alcoholics than among the general population.

It is interesting that certain types of cancers seem strongly linked to specific types of alcoholic beverages. For example, cancer of the esophagus is associated with drinking a native Japanese beverage called shochu, with African maize beer, with wine in Normandy and with pai-kan, a strong beverage made in China. In Puerto Rico esophageal cancer is thought to be caused by illicitly distilled rum, while beer made in Hawaii has been linked to eight types of cancer. In the United States, colon and rectal cancer have been associated with beer drinking. Although animal tests have shown that alcohol itself may be a carcinogen, the examples above seem to suggest that alcohol's primary role in cancer formation might be promoting the activity of other chemical carcinogens found in specific beverages and associated with specific types of cancers.

Among the cancer-causing agents in alcoholic beverages are aflatoxin, a natural toxin known to cause liver cancer; fusel oil, a substance produced when certain fruits and vegetables are distilled; benzo(a)pyrene; asbestos fibers (contaminants from filters used to clarify wine, beer and gin); and nitrosamines. The presence of nitrosamines in American beers and whiskeys produced a heated controversy when it was first disclosed in 1979. Since then, better manufacturing methods have eliminated much of the nitrosamine content of these beverages, but amounts up to several parts per billion may still be present. Less widely known is the fact that most wines have been shown to be mutagenic in biological tests. The mutagenic agents may be pesticides and other chemicals used in the growing of grapes or other substances and chemicals introduced during the fermentation and bottling of wine.

The cancer-promoting, and possibly cancer-inducing, effects of alcohol are enhanced by smoking, a troubling fact in light of the tendency of heavy drinkers to also be heavy smokers. Among heavy drinkers who do not smoke and heavy smokers who do not drink, the risk of developing mouth or pharynx cancer is two to three times the risk for nondrinkers and nonsmokers. For those who both drink and smoke heavily, though, the risk is 15 times greater. It is thought that the carcinogens in cigarette smoke initiate cancers, while the alcohol promotes their development. This relationship is believed to hold for other cancers of the head and neck areas, making those who both smoke and drink heavily at particularly high risk to cancer.

Giving up just heavy drinking or just heavy smoking will markedly reduce one's risk from head and neck cancers. Of course, it is best to reduce or eliminate one's indulgence in both habits, but if a heavy drinker and smoker were to give up just one-half of his or her dual addiction it should be smoking as far as cancer risk is concerned. About 22 percent of all cancers and 33 percent of cancer deaths in men are due to lung cancer. Oral cancer, on the other hand, accounts for only 5 percent of cancers and 3 percent of cancer deaths.

The health effects of alcohol are partly caused by the poor nutrition of many alcoholics. Many alcoholics substitute the calories in alcohol for the calories in food. In addition, alcohol itself can contribute to poor nutrition by interfering with the absorption and utilization of vitamins. The alcoholic's poor blood-clotting ability can be pinned on a reduced absorption of vitamin K, for example. Alcohol's interference with the utilization of beta-carotene from vegetables can cause an inadequate vitamin A intake. Osteoporosis, or brittle bones, among alcoholics is caused by alcohol's prevention of the normal utilization of vitamin D. Nutritional deficiencies, especially a deficiency of vitamin A, may also contribute to the alcoholic's risk of head and neck cancers.

The most common and serious deficiency caused by heavy

drinking is that of the B vitamins. Lack of B vitamins has been strongly linked with another affliction of alcoholics, polyneuritis. Sufferers of this disorder experience painful inflammation of nerves in various parts of the body. Polyneuritis can be caused by a blow to the body, bone fractures and penetrating injuries, but a leading cause is the malnutrition brought on by alcoholism.

That polyneuritis can be caused by a poor diet has been suspected for many years. In 1933 a researcher, noting that beriberi, a syndrome caused by a B vitamin deficiency, and polyneuritis were often seen together, speculated that polyneuritis was also caused by a lack of B vitamins. Work later in that decade and in the 1940s showed that supplements of vitamin B could reduce the incidence of polyneuritis in affected alcoholics, confirming the link between the nutrient and the disorder.

Eventually, thiamine, or vitamin B_1, was found to be the specific member of the B family responsible for preventing the neurologic symptoms. It is not surprising that alcoholics often have thiamine deficiencies, which stem from their generally poor nutrition, their reduced ability to absorb the vitamin through the digestive tract and their tendency to eliminate it more quickly than the average person. Alcohol also seems to block the process by which the body converts thiamine to its active forms. So the thiamine that is absorbed by alcoholics may ultimately not be useful. In addition, heavy drinkers store less thiamine in the liver than most people.

Pyridoxine is another B vitamin that is often in short supply in the bodies of alcoholics. A deficiency of this vitamin may contribute to the development of cirrhosis. Without sufficient pyridoxine, liver cells tend to become fatty, a condition that resembles the early stages of cirrhosis. And, without pyridoxine, the body is unable to protect liver cells from the damaging effects of alcohol, and the liver is unable to maintain a rapid enough rate of cell division to replace liver cells destroyed by alcohol.

The mineral zinc seems able to protect the liver from alcohol. Zinc is a component of an enzyme that breaks down alcohol into other compounds prior to its excretion by the kidneys. In experiments with mice and rats, supplements of zinc drastically reduced the mortality rate after the administration of large doses of alcohol. Unfortunately, most heavy drinkers have low blood-serum levels of zinc. One way to reduce the incidence of liver disease among alcoholics might be to add zinc supplements to beer, wine and other alcoholic beverages.

Other nutrients that should be considered as additives for alcoholic beverages are vitamin C and sulfur-containing amino acids. Together, these nutrients have proved able to protect the body against the effects of acetaldehyde, a chemical produced when alcohol is metabolized in the liver. Also found in the blood of cigarette smokers, acetaldehyde is more poisonous than alcohol itself and has been associated with alcoholic cardiomyopathy, a disease of the heart muscle, and alcohol addiction. It is believed that vitamin C does not act directly on acetaldehyde, but rather helps the liver destroy alcohol without producing acetaldehyde by protecting a compound called nicotinamide adenine dinucleotide (NAD), which is required for the metabolism of alcohol. Vitamin C may also help eliminate alcohol from the body, thereby reducing the amount that can be converted to acetaldehyde.

It is unfortunate that heavy drinkers, those most susceptible to acetaldehyde and the many other toxic and carcinogenic substances in alcohol, are often the least prepared, from a nutritional standpoint, to protect themselves from these substances. The abuse of alcohol is all too often accompanied by moderately to extremely poor nutrition. It seems imperative that programs designed to help alcoholics overcome their drinking problems should also help them get the nourishment needed to fight off the hazards in alcohol. Such a program should focus on encouraging alcoholics to consume a diet rich in B vitamins, in particular B_1 or thiamine, which helps prevent polyneuritis, and pyridoxine, which may help prevent cirrhosis. The alcoholic's diet should also include good sources of zinc, vitamin C and protein (a source of sulfur-containing amino acids), as these nutrients seem to protect the liver from the ravages of alcohol.

FIBER: THE LIFESAVER IN OUR FOOD

Each year about 100,000 Americans are diagnosed as having cancer of the colon. Colon cancer accounts for nearly 15 percent of all diagnosed cancers and a similar percentage of all cancer deaths. It has been called one of the most life-threatening of all cancers, because unless it is detected in its early stages, the prognosis is unusually grim. In the last 40 years, evidence has accumulated to suggest that diet can be both a cause and a preventer of colon cancer. This section will deal with how diet can lower the incidence of colon cancer; the next will detail how diet can contribute to its occurrence.

In 1950, evidence first appeared suggesting that a component of the diet known as fiber might prevent cancers of the colon and rectum. Two researchers fed rats diets containing either three or six percent crude fiber and then exposed them to small quantities of a potent carcinogen known as acetyl amino fluorine, or AAF. Rats raised on the higher-fiber diet had considerably fewer cancers of the colon than the animals fed the low-fiber diet. Since then, several encouraging studies have demonstrated that a number of cancer-causing agents, among them DDT, PCBs, heavy metals and x-rays, are less likely to cause lower-digestive-tract cancers in animals fed a high-fiber diet. In these studies, the higher the level of fiber fed to animals, the lower the number of tumors that resulted.

Fiber is usually defined as plant matter that is not capable of being digested in the human gastrointestinal tract. Among the common components of fiber (the amount and type varying with the kind of food) are pectin, a complex sugar found primarily in fruit; cellulose, a long chain of glucose molecules that makes plant stems rigid; lignins, which make up the skeletons of plants; waxes; brans; germs; husks; and naturally occurring gums. Certain food additives, such as synthetic gums and methylcellulose, also add fiber to the diet.

As a population, Americans consume considerably less fiber than many other cultures. Dennis Burkett, a British scientist, was curious about how this difference in fiber consumption correlated with colon cancer rates. In 1972 he published a study that compared the health of a British population consuming a typical low-fiber, high-fat Western diet with that of an African population, which consumes as much as five times more fiber. The African villagers, Burkett found, had a markedly lower incidence of lower digestive tract cancers.

To date, not enough evidence has been gathered to say conclu-

TABLE 5 | GOOD SOURCES OF FIBER

Food	Serving	Crude Fiber Content (grams)*
Apple, with skin	1 medium	2.3
Apricots, dried	1 cup	2.4
Apricots, dehydrated	4 oz.	4.3
Avocado	1 fruit	16.4
Black beans	4 oz.	5.0
Blackberries, hulled	½ cup	3.0
Broccoli, boiled	1 medium stalk	2.7
Brussels sprouts, boiled	1 cup	2.5
Black walnuts, shelled	4 oz.	1.9
Chestnuts	4 oz.	1.2
Chick peas	½ cup	5.0
Coconut meat	4 oz.	4.5
Crude bran	1 oz.	2.6
Dates, pitted	4 oz.	2.6
Elderberries	4 oz.	7.9
Figs, dried	½ cup	4.8
Green beans, boiled	½ cup	0.6
Green peas, boiled	½ cup	1.6
Kidney beans, cooked	½ cup	1.4
Lentils, cooked	½ cup	1.2
Lima beans, boiled	½ cup	1.6
Parsnips, pared	4 oz.	2.3
Pear	1 medium	2.3
Raspberries	½ cup	3.4
Roasted peanuts, chopped	½ cup	1.7
Soybeans, boiled	4 oz.	7.6
Turnip, boiled	½ cup	1.0
Whole wheat bread	2 slices	0.8
Whole wheat crackers	1 oz.	0.9

Fiber analysis by the U.S. Department of Agriculture

* Crude fiber analysis tends to miss much of the fiber naturally present in food, and is therefore only a rough measure of the actual fiber content of food. The foods in this table may have at least five times the amount of fiber indicated.

sively how fiber prevents colon and rectal cancers, but several theories have been offered. It has been suggested, for example, that fiber may dilute the carcinogenic agents in food, or bind with them, keeping them away from the wall of the bowel and lowering the chance that they might initiate a cancer. A more widely accepted theory is that fiber retains water, which softens the stool and eases its passage through the large intestine. With a more rapid transit time, the waste material and any cancer-causing agents in it have less time to make contact with the tissue of the colon and rectum and less time to cause a cancer.

If it is true that Americans eat too little fiber, then how much is enough? Most experts agree this question is difficult to answer as yet, though many say that the average American could probably stand to double his or her intake. This should bring the amount of dietary fiber consumed to approximately what a typical vegetarian eats, or about 30 to 40 grams a day. Table 5 lists some foods that are good sources of fiber.

It is best to increase one's intake of fiber gradually and not overdo it in an attempt to avoid colon cancer. And it is important to remember that a high-fiber diet (as opposed to an adequate-fiber diet) does have risks. The most important is the ability of fiber to hinder the gastrointestinal absorption of vital nutrients. Just as fiber in the diet reduces the amount of time that carcinogens are in contact with the digestive tract, it also lowers the amount of time that nutrients can be captured. For most people, the reduced nutrient uptake poses little or no risk, but for the elderly, the poorly nourished and adolescents, whose nutrition is often already inadequate, adding appreciable amounts of fiber to the diet can cause malnutrition. Fiber can also cause gas, a bloated feeling and diarrhea, problems that can be reduced if fiber is added gradually to the diet.

Two fiber-pollutant interactions should be mentioned here, both because they have been well supported by research and because they have important public health implications:

Strontium and Alginate

Strontium 90 is a heavy radioactive element that has been an infrequent threat to public health. To date, most of the strontium

90 in the environment has come from the above-ground detonation of nuclear weapons. Although an international nuclear test ban treaty has reduced the number of above-ground explosions, clouds of radioactive fallout laced with strontium have traveled across the United States on several occasions in recent history after test detonations in the People's Republic of China.

Strontium 90 is a well-known and powerful cancer-causing agent that is readily assimilated by bones. With a half-life of 28 years and a tendency to act like calcium in the food chain, strontium is absorbed by plants and animals, concentrated in cow's milk and, ultimately, assimilated by the human body.

A fiber derived from kelp, a common brown seaweed, has been found to prevent strontium-90–induced cancers by selectively inhibiting the absorption of strontium through the digestive tract. The substance, called sodium alginate, has proven in tests to lower the blood and bone levels of strontium 90 in rats without affecting the absorption of calcium or normal digestion.

Alginate can be made into a jellylike substance that is palatable to people. In fact, it is already being used in fast-food milkshakes and some instant puddings. Work with human subjects has shown that supplements should prevent the absorption of strontium 90 through the human digestive tract. In one study, just a gram and a half of alginate caused a tenfold reduction in strontium uptake. Encouraged by these initial findings, scientists have attempted to see if alginate would act in a similar way with lead, a serious health threat to young children. Unfortunately, alginate seems to have no effect on lead uptake in humans and actually increases its absorption in rats, which will probably limit its utility for humans except when exposure to fallout from nuclear-weapons tests is imminent.

Lead and Pectate

While alginate has no effect on lead absorption, pectate, a fiber derived from fruits, has been found to reduce lead uptake by nearly 90 percent in laboratory animals and to lower lead levels in the blood, kidney and liver. As we noted in Chapter 6, several Soviet researchers were able to greatly reduce the lead-induced changes in red blood cells in lead workers by administering apple pectin to the workers every day. The results of this and other research suggest that pectin may be a potent weapon in the fight against lead poisoning in children, which is now estimated to affect about four percent of all preschool-aged kids.

FAT, FADS AND CANCER

In the previous section, we noted that the consumption of fiber can reduce one's risk of cancer of the lower digestive tract. But it has become clear in recent years that fiber is not the only dietary constituent that may play a key role in the development of cancer. Fat, a component of the diet that Americans tend to eat too much of, has been linked with cancers of the colon, breast, uterus, prostate gland and other tissues.

Epidemiologists have noticed that the incidence of colon cancer in Japan is considerably lower than the rate in the United States. When Japanese emigrate to the United States, their risk of colon cancer rises gradually and ultimately becomes about equal to that of the average American by the third or fourth generation. Likewise, the breast cancer rate among Japanese-American women is more than double the rate for women in Japan. On the other hand, in this country the incidence of breast cancer among Seventh-Day Adventist women, many of whom are vegetarians, is one-half to two-thirds that of the general population of adult women.

The reason for the lower cancer incidence among the Japanese and Seventh-Day Adventists seems to be diet, and in particular, fats. Following a more traditional Eastern diet, both of these groups consume considerably less fried food and other fats. There are undoubtedly other factors that lower their cancer risk (see *A Lifestyle to Emulate* below), but fat intake is easily one of the most important.

Fats are believed to be promoters rather than initiators of cancer. In the case of colon cancer, for example, it is believed that fat may promote the activity of carcinogens normally found in the feces and stimulate bacteria in the colon to convert bile and various steroids into carcinogenic substances, which can then act on the lining of the lower bowel and initiate cancer.

The relationship between fat and breast cancer is a bit more complicated. The initiation and progression of this disease seem to be related to the quantity of estrogen a woman produces during adolescence and adult life. In particular, the ratio of a type of estrogen known as estriol, or E_3, to the two other estrogens normally found in the female body seems to strongly influence one's risk of developing breast cancer. The higher the ratio of E_3 to the other two estrogens, it is believed, the lower the risk of breast cancer. Interestingly, a pregnancy early in life lowers a woman's risk of breast cancer. This is probably related to the fact that during pregnancy, a woman's estrogen production increases, with elevated estriol output accounting for most of the increase.

It is believed that fats lower the ratio of E_3 to the other estrogens in the female body. The greater the amount of fat in the diet, the lower the ratio. The other estrogens may interact with fats to promote the activity of chemical carcinogens. So the more fat and the greater the ratio of the other estrogens to E_3, the greater the risk of breast cancer, the theory goes. Supporting this theory is the fact that breast cancer is strongly linked with early menarche or obesity during adolescence, the period when many breast cancers are believed to be initiated. Both early menarche and obesity can be caused by eating a high fat diet. It is also interesting to note that Japanese women, who consume fewer fats than American women, have a higher ratio of E_3 to the other estrogens and a considerably lower incidence of breast cancer.

The link between fats and both chemical carcinogenesis and toxicity has been under study since the turn of the century. The toxicity or carcinogenicity of over 20 chemical agents is now known to be affected by fats and the list is expected to grow. In most cases, fats enhance the effects of carcinogens and toxins on the body, though for two chemicals, the natural poison aflatoxin and the explosive TNT, fats do offer some protection against the onset of cancer and intoxication, respectively.

Among the more interesting interactions are these:

—When fats and fluoride are present together in the stomach, the stomach takes more time to empty its contents into the small intestine. This may result in a greater rate of absorption of fluoride and a greater body burden of this mineral, which has been linked to mottling of the teeth in children (see Chapter 6).

—Bile salts and phospholipids secreted into the digestive tract to aid in the digestion of fats seem to enhance the absorption of lead. Some researchers have suggested that lead workers be encouraged to eat a low-fat diet.

—In a controlled study, rats on a high-fat diet developed considerably more tumors of the mammary glands than rats on a low-fat diet when exposed to diethylstilbestrol (DES).

—Some research suggests that the number of leukemialike changes in the blood in animals exposed to the carcinogen benzene increases as the amount of fat in the diet increases.

Several researchers have noted that it is not just the amount of fat in the diet that raises one's risk of cancer. Quality is also important. Fats that contain unsaturated or polyunsaturated fatty acids seem much more likely to enhance the activity of carcinogens than fats with a high proportion of saturated fatty acids. Saturation refers to the number of double bonds or links between the carbon atoms in the long chains of fatty acids, one component of fat molecules. A fatty acid is saturated if it has no double bonds, unsaturated if it has one double bond and polyunsaturated if more than one.

In 1971, M. L. Pearce and S. Dayton took a second look at a group of people who had participated in an eight-year study of the effects of saturated and polyunsaturated fats on the development of coronary heart disease. Several such studies have shown that diets high in saturated fats may spur the development of heart disease. In their reexamination, which was published in the prestigious British medical journal *Lancet,* they found that, although the incidence of heart disease was lower, deaths from cancer were considerably higher in the group that had consumed diets high in polyunsaturated fatty acids. This confirmed many similar findings obtained in work with animals.

Just how unsaturated fatty acids predispose one to developing cancer is not known. It has been suggested that large amounts of polyunsaturated fats may inhibit the immunological system, which is believed to squash new cancers before they are able to progress. It is also thought that cell membranes that have a high proportion of polyunsaturated fats may be more likely to allow carcinogens into the cell where they can damage DNA.

However they act, news about the cancer-promoting effect of polyunsaturated fatty acids leaves Americans with a dilemma.

Many Americans have already replaced many of the saturated fats in their diets, such as butter, with polyunsaturated fats, such as margarine. However, that choice may place them at an increased risk to the effects of chemical carcinogens. How to solve this dilemma is a matter for each individual to decide, based on his or her risk from heart disease and cancer. If you have a family history of heart or vascular disease, a diet that favors unsaturated fats would probably be the best choice. Likewise, if you are overweight, smoke or have a high serum cholesterol count, you should probably stay away from saturated fats. On the other hand, if you have a high incidence in your family of certain types of cancer, such as cancer of the colon, or if you work around chemicals that are known carcinogens, a diet that includes principally saturated fats might lower your risk of cancer. Whether the fats you eat are saturated or unsaturated, you should probably try to lower your overall intake of fats to help prevent obesity, heart disease and cancer.

While the problem for most Americans is eating too much fat, some Americans occasionally eat too little. When it is put on a prolonged fast, the body may begin breaking down its stores of fat to get energy. Unfortunately, several known toxins and carcinogens are stored in body fat. While locked in the fat, they are relatively harmless. However, if the fats are broken down, the poisons can leave the fatty deposits and enter the bloodstream. Once in the blood, they can travel to sites in the body where they can cause tissue damage.

That this can happen was demonstrated by K. L. Davison and his colleagues at North Dakota State University. Davison raised chickens on a feed that was mixed with various quantities (up to 20 parts per million) of a chlorinated pesticide known as dieldrin. The feed was then cut off and the animals observed as they were slowly starved over the next few weeks. As the body weight of the chickens dropped, evidence that body fat was being broken down, the level of pesticides in the chickens' blood rapidly rose and a few of the chickens actually died from dieldrin poisoning.

Whether starvation in humans could result in pesticide poisoning is not known, although increases in blood pesticide levels have been observed after rapid weight loss in people. The risk would probably be greatest among farmers, gardeners, insecticide workers and others who are likely to be exposed to pesticides on a regular basis. However, because of the lack of evidence to support the effectiveness of crash weight loss programs, there is probably no reason for anyone to fast and risk possible pesticide intoxication.

CONCLUSION: A LIFESTYLE TO EMULATE

If you took the advice of the previous sections seriously, you should by now be thinking about quitting smoking, cutting down on your drinking and eating more fiber, and you should also be considering the quantity and quality of the fats you eat. Seventh-Day Adventists, members of a Christian faith who observe the Sabbath on Saturday, already follow these guidelines. They do not smoke or drink and most follow an ovo-lacto-vegetarian regime, meaning that they do not eat meat, but do consume eggs and certain dairy products. Of those who do eat meat, most abstain from pork and all do not drink coffee or tea or use hot condiments or spices.

Not surprisingly, in a study of over 35,000 Seventh-Day Adventists carried out between 1958 and 1965, they were found to have a longer life expectancy than the rest of the United States population and a cancer death rate one-half to one-third as great as that of the general population. Cancers with a particularly low incidence in this group include those associated with smoking and drinking, such as lung and esophageal cancer as well as others linked to dietary factors like colon and breast cancers.

That diet plays a role in the lower cancer risk among Seventh-Day Adventists was demonstrated in a study of breast and colon cancer patients in a Seventh-Day Adventists' hospital. It was found that the colon cancer cases were associated with the consumption of beef, lamb and other high-fat foods as well as the heavy use of dairy products (except milk). The findings were less conclusive for breast cancer, though the use of fried foods was found to increase a woman's risk. In all cases, eating green leafy vegetables, vegetable protein product and vegetables high in fiber were negatively correlated with the risk of cancer.

Despite its benefits, many people will likely choose not to follow the ascetic way of the Seventh-Day Adventists. Some will accept the risk inherent in a moderate- or high-fat diet or a diet low in fiber in order to enjoy those foods the Adventists would avoid. Others will continue to smoke, again accepting a sizable risk in order to continue a behavior they find pleasurable. And some will continue to drink heavily, perhaps unwilling or unable to cease this destructive behavior.

What this chapter has shown is that we can often control the magnitude of the risks we choose to accept. Just as we can wear seat belts when we drive a car or install an adequate ventilation system in a brick house, we can reduce our risk from cancer and other serious diseases by giving some consideration to what we eat. As noted above, how much fiber and fat we eat can influence our susceptibility to colon cancer. Fat consumption may also affect our chances of getting breast cancer. The research to date strongly indicates that Americans may be able to lower their risk of cancer by increasing their intake of fiber and lowering their consumption of fat.

With regard to fiber, it is best to not increase one's intake too quickly. If you choose a high-fiber regime, begin with just a bit more fiber than you now consume. Try adding a high-fiber cereal or a whole-grain bread. Gradually increase your fiber content to about twice what you now consume, using the table in this chapter as a guide to good sources of fiber. Parents who suspect their children may be exposed to higher-than-average amounts of lead, for example families who live near a major highway or in a city, should consider giving their children more fruit each day, for example an additional apple or two, since the pectin in fruit can decrease the absorption of lead.

As far as fat goes, to reduce one's risk of cancer one should eat a diet low in fats, according to research described in this chapter. In particular, lowering one's consumption of unsaturated fats, the kind found in margarine and corn oil, has been found to lower cancer risk in animal tests. However, the consumption of saturated fats has been linked to heart disease. So, whether one chooses to consume primarily unsaturated or saturated fats depends on whether one has a family history of cancer or heart disease.

While diets with excess fat seem to promote cancer, another nutrient in excess, vitamin A, has shown great promise as a potential anticancer agent. Experiments with animals have shown that large doses of vitamin A can prevent, and even cure, cancer. However, the doses necessary to prevent cancer in people would be poisonous. Work is now underway with synthetic forms of vitamin A that may be more effective and less toxic than the natural vitamin. Evidence from a major epidemiological study has suggested that a form of vitamin A known as carotene may work to prevent cancers at levels normally found in the human diet. The study found that workers at a telephone plant who had eaten the highest levels of carotene had the lowest rate of lung cancer. The results applied even to workers who smoked. The study indicated that people who, despite frequent warnings, continue to smoke may be able to lower their risk of cancer simply by eating plenty of yellow, orange and leafy green vegetables, all good sources of carotene.

Smokers can protect themselves from two toxic components of smoke, cyanide and cadmium, through nutrition. Evidence indicates that the dimness of vision occasionally seen in cigarette smokers may be an overt sign of cyanide poisoning. Supplements of vitamin B_{12} have been effective in curing this condition, known as tobacco amblyopia. Long-term exposure to cadmium in cigarette smoke is believed to be related to the development of emphysema. The presence of cadmium causes a deficiency of a chemical known as serum-alpha-1-antitrypsin. This deficiency allows an enzyme known as trypsin to damage lung cells. Zinc and vitamins C and E may help the body deactivate and get rid of the cadmium in cigarette smoke.

The smoking of cigarettes is a major health problem in the United States. Another common threat to good health is heavy drinking. The abuse of alcohol has been associated with a variety of liver disorders, including cirrhosis and liver cancer. In addition, heavy drinkers have a high risk of cancers of the esophagus, larynx, pharynx and mouth, possibly because of a variety of chemical carcinogens known to be in certain alcoholic beverages. Many alcoholics do not eat adequate diets, an unfortunate fact in light of evidence that certain nutrients may help alleviate the ravages of alcohol. In particular, zinc, vitamin C and protein may all help prevent the cell damage and cancer that alcohol is known to promote, vitamin B_1 seems to be important in preventing polyneuritis, and pyridoxine may help head off cirrhosis of the liver.

CHAPTER 10

Summing Up: More Questions than Answers

In the preceding chapters, we have assessed the current notion that nutrition can alter your susceptibility to environmentally induced sickness. We have found that in many respects this notion does, in fact, have a legitimate and scientific basis. Time after time, research has shown that diets deficient in various nutrients (in other words, diets that have less than the Recommended Dietary Allowance, or RDA, of vitamins, minerals or other nutrients) can markedly enhance the toxicity of a wide variety of environmental contaminants. Though it is not nearly as often the case, we have found examples of protection from pollutants offered by doses of nutrients consumed in excess of dietary requirements. We have also noted that some nutrients, most notably fats, when consumed in excess can greatly increase the odds that you will be the victim of hazards in the environment.

Several important questions would seem to remain. How can one use all of this information to lead a safer, healthier life? What is the bottom line on nutrient-pollutant interactions? What should one eat or avoid in order to hold the harmful agents in the environment at bay? Just what is the ultimate, perfect, ideal diet?

Unfortunately, the jury is still out on these questions. As far as we have come in the study of nutrition, there are still far too many questions to answer, far too many hypotheses to test and far too many studies to be conducted. The answers we as a society need will not appear overnight. It will take years of research, much of it very expensive, before firm recommendations can be made.

191

That elusive ideal diet is like a jigsaw puzzle with only a few of the pieces in place. The pieces that are already there are extremely encouraging. The evidence emerging from the study of nutrient-pollutant interactions indicates that a proper diet may be an extremely useful tool with which people can ward off environmental disease. In fact, it is quite possible that nutrition may one day do for cancer and other environmental ills what fluoridation has done for dental health in this country. Good nutrition will probably never eliminate environmental disease, but it may markedly lower its incidence at a very small cost to society.

It is likely that we will enter the next century with many pieces of the puzzle yet to be filled in. This creates a natural conflict between scientists and government regulators on the one hand and the public on the other. Scientists and regulators, who are charged with finding answers about nutrition and setting our national nutrition policies, like to be sure of things before they pronounce them to be true and useful. If it takes years to determine beyond a reasonable doubt that the Recommended Dietary Allowances should be increased, so be it.

Most people, understandably, want answers now. Every day they spend waiting for guidance means another day of exposure to the myriad substances and agents in the environment that can make them sick. If scientists and government regulators don't provide this guidance, there are many others who are more than willing to fill the information gap, often with questionable advice.

We have attempted to provide answers, where they exist. But often, as we have seen, the answers are just not there or are just not good enough. Not yet. By far the majority of work on the relationship between diet and pollution has been done with animals, and much of that with animals as distant from man as mice and guinea pigs. The art of extrapolation from animal results to human experience is still imprecise at best. So, while a great deal of the work we have described is promising, even tantalizing, it is still in need of verification with human studies.

But there are certain things that we do know right now. There are, in fact, relationships that are clear-cut and that can be applied today. The first of these is quite simple. In a great many of the cases described in this book, it has been shown that deficiencies of certain nutrients increase one's susceptibility to the toxic and carcinogenic chemicals around us. So, an easy way to increase one's resistance to the environment is to eat a balanced diet. That may sound like unnecessary advice, but surprising as it seems, many Americans do not get all the nutrients they need.

We tend to think of the United States as a land of plenty and of Americans as generally healthy and well nourished. It is hard to believe that, in a nation that exports so much food, nutritional deficiencies are common. Millions of Americans do not eat the Recommended Dietary Allowances of one or more nutrients. Many are deficient in two or more nutrients. Children, the elderly and menstruating, pregnant or nursing women are the most likely to have deficiencies because of their increased need for many nutrients, but nutritional deficiencies have been found in all types of people, regardless of age, sex, race or income.

For instance, several government nutrition surveys in recent years have determined that nine out of ten black children aged one to five who live below the poverty level consume less than the RDA of iron. Nearly half of those children do not get their dietary requirement of vitamins A and C and about a third do not eat enough calcium. The story is about the same for poor white children, the one exception being that only 15 percent of poor whites are deficient in calcium.

Surprisingly, about the same percentages of black and white children above the poverty line do not consume the dietary requirement for these four nutrients. Of particular concern is the fact that people do not seem to eat better diets as they grow older. Adults in all income classes are likely to suffer from nutritional deficiencies. Women are the worst offenders. About 95 percent of women sampled in the government surveys consumed less than the RDA of iron. The percentage of women deficient in vitamins A and C ranged from about 40 percent for white women living above the poverty level to about 70 percent for poor white women.

What this means is that there are millions of Americans, rich and poor, whose diets are inadequate by government standards. And the major finding of literally hundreds of animal studies is that inadequate diets—often just marginally inadequate—may markedly increase the toxicity of a wide range of heavy metals, especially lead and cadmium, synthetic organic chemicals, and other agents known to be toxic or carcinogenic.

The easiest way to get the nutrients one needs would be to take nutrient supplements, such as vitamin or mineral pills. But before you look to pills to boost your diet, look at your diet. The key to good nutrition is not in a bottle, but on your dinner plate. Try to eat a balanced diet, with generous and regular portions of green, leafy green, yellow and orange vegetables as well as citrus fruits, adequate carbohydrates, whole-grain products and not too much fat. Chapter 3 lists good sources of many of the important nutrients. While this regime may not offer you complete protection from the environment, the evidence strongly suggests that the vitamins, minerals and proteins in a balanced diet will go a long way toward increasing your resistance to environmental disease.

If you absolutely cannot eat a balanced diet, for example if you eat a lot of fast food or do not always consume enough vegetables or fruit, you may be one of the millions of Americans who are at least marginally deficient in one or more nutrients. A multi-vitamin and mineral supplement, one that contains just a portion of the Recommended Dietary Allowance for several nutrients, might be right for you. Vitamin and mineral supplements are also appropriate for pregnant and nursing women, postoperative patients and vegetarians (who may need to take vitamin B_{12} supplements).

The importance of adequate nutrition becomes dramatically clear when one considers the number of hazardous agents that become even more toxic or more carcinogenic when introduced into a body that has been poorly nourished. We have cited many such examples in this book. Here is a summary of some of the most important ones:

—In animal tests deficiencies of vitamin A and the B vitamin pyridoxine have increased the toxicity of aflatoxin, a natural poison produced by a fungus that lives on peanuts and other nuts and grains and is commonly found in peanut butter.

—Deficiencies of zinc or the B vitamins may place you at an increased risk to the carcinogenic effects of nitrosamines, strong cancer-causing substances produced when chemicals known as amines combine with sodium nitrite, a coloring agent and preservative used in many cured meats and smoked fish.

—A deficiency of vitamin C may elevate one's risk of suffering the toxic effects of the common environmental pollutant DDT.

—Deficiencies of calcium, phosphorus, copper, magnesium, iron, vitamin C and vitamin E may enhance the toxicity of the pervasive heavy metal lead. Consuming too little of these nutrients, especially the five minerals, could elevate a child's risk of brain damage as well as the other toxic effects of lead.

—Animal tests have shown that too little zinc, calcium or vitamin C can increase the toxicity of another common heavy metal, cadmium.

—Consuming insufficient vitamin E may make the lining of the respiratory tract more vulnerable to the damage done by the common air pollutants ozone and nitrogen dioxide.

Exposure to certain pollutants and drugs will very likely increase your requirements for various nutrients, making a balanced diet all the more important. For example, chlorinated organic chemicals, such as PCBs and the pesticide DDT, seem to increase one's requirement for vitamin A. Many industrial chemicals may increase the dietary requirements for certain nutrients, and in fact even marginal deficiencies of these nutrients often greatly increase the effects of these chemicals in experiments with animals. Many chemicals, including arsenic, chromium, silica, tellurium, and benzene, increase the body's need for vitamin C. Carbon tetrachloride and carbon disulfide may increase one's need for B vitamins and repeated exposure to loud noise may elevate one's requirements for vitamins A and C.

If you smoke a pack or more of cigarettes a day, you probably need more vitamin C than a nonsmoker. A glass of orange juice or a 100-milligram tablet should fill your daily requirement. It is also generally agreed that heavy drinkers may need extra thiamine, pyridoxine and zinc. While the jury is still out on the additional nutritional requirements of users of oral contraceptives, several researchers have suggested that women on the pill have an increased need for vitamin B_6. One researcher has suggested that pill users take 30 milligrams of B_6 every day, which is 15 times the RDA for adult women. Whether oral contraceptives actually increase a woman's need for vitamin B_6 to that extent is not known, but the evidence does indicate that many women on the pill do need more than the RDA of B_6.

There is disagreement as to whether the use of large doses of aspirin by rheumatoid arthritis patients increases their need for vitamin C, although the data seem to support this conclusion. There is also evidence from animal studies and some work with people that other drugs increase the body's need for various nutrients. Anticonvulsant medications used by many people who suffer from epilepsy seem to be capable of causing serious shortages of vitamin D. Laxatives, antacids and broad-spectrum antibiotics can cause deficiencies of several nutrients. On the other hand, oral contraceptives, in addition to causing a B vitamin deficiency, may also cause the body to retain excess calcium and vitamins A and K.

Though the research we have looked at does suggest that people who fall into the categories mentioned above need nutritional supplements, the evidence does not support the use of extremely large doses of nutrients to reduce the adverse effects of pollutants. In some cases, the toxic or carcinogenic effects of certain environmental agents have been prevented or lessened in animal trials with large doses of nutrients, but the doses of the chemicals under study and the nutrients being evaluated were often many times higher than what would have been safe for a human being, which makes drawing conclusions very difficult. As was pointed out in Chapter 3, very large doses of vitamin A and several minerals are themselves toxic. Therefore, we feel that so-called megadoses of these nutrients are potentially dangerous and that the dangers probably outweigh any benefit that they may hold in the fight against pollution. In any case, a great deal more research, especially with human subjects, must be done to resolve this issue.

This does not mean, however, that one should never eat more than the RDA of any particular nutrient. As we pointed out earlier, smokers, oral contraceptive users, heavy drinkers and others may in fact need supplements of certain nutrients. What this does mean is that most studies of nutrient-pollutant interactions have focused on the effects of nutritional deficiencies and not on discovering whether levels of nutrients in excess of the RDAs can offer protection. Consequently, there is far less information on this type of interaction. Nevertheless, there are a few nutrients that we can recommend that you consume in excess of dietary requirements, or more accurately we believe that any potential risk from taking supplements of these nutrients is far outweighed by the benefits such supplements may bring.

First, if you eat preserved meats (cured ham, bacon, cold cuts, and so on), smoked fish or other foods that contain nitrites, you should drink orange juice or eat an orange or two along with each meal that includes these foods. The best strategy is to consume the juice or fruit just before your meal, so the vitamin C will be waiting in the stomach ready to prevent the formation of cancer-causing nitrosamines. A cup of orange juice or two oranges will give you in one dose up to two times the RDA for vitamin C, but this type of supplementation is quite safe and very beneficial.

The results of tests of the cancer-fighting ability of vitamin A in animals have been encouraging and suggest that supplements of this vitamin may also be beneficial. Unfortunately, the doses of vitamin A used in experiments done to date would be toxic to people. Work is underway with synthetic vitamin A molecules, which are less toxic than natural vitamin A, and which may offer greater protection against cancer. Though these manmade vitamins are now being tested in trials with human subjects to see if they can indeed prevent or cure cancers, it will probably be years before they are available to the public, assuming they are proven to be effective.

In the meantime, we can recommend that you eat plenty of vegetables, especially the yellow, orange and leafy green varieties. Just as high levels of vitamin A may prevent cancer, a deficiency of this vitamin can increase your risk to this life-threatening disease. A growing number of studies employing a large number of human subjects in several countries have found that the dietary level of carotene, the form of vitamin A found in vegetables, is inversely related to the occurrence of lung and digestive tract cancers. However these human studies have not proved that a diet high in carotene reduces the risk of cancer. Technically, all they have established is that high carotene intake and low cancer incidence are related. The best scientific minds, both in and out of government, believe that more work is needed before a cause and effect relationship can be established.

Nevertheless, since carotene is not known to be toxic to humans even at high levels and since the body of available evidence strongly suggests that it may lower the risk of cancer, we recommend that Americans consume diets that have rich sources of carotene every day, even if this means eating more than the RDA for vitamin A. In particular, smokers, industrial workers exposed to carcinogenic substances such as asbestos, coke oven emissions and many organic chemicals, and anyone constantly exposed to automobile exhaust, woodstove smoke or other known carcinogenic agents may lower their cancer risk by 30 to 70 percent by eating a high-carotene diet, based on the results of the human studies conducted so far. So, while carotene is not a proven cancer preventer, making sure your diet is rich in this nutrient can't hurt.

Fiber is another dietary component that may play a role in preventing cancers and that most Americans probably eat too little of. Evidence from several epidemiological studies as well as from work with animals has shown that the level of fiber in the diet is related to the risk of cancer of the lower digestive tract. The rate of colon cancer, in fact, is lower among vegetarians and in cultures that consume a great deal of fiber than among most Americans who consume the typical Western low-fiber diet. There is not enough evidence yet to establish any sort of Recommended Dietary Allowance for fiber, but many researchers say that the average American could probably stand to double his or her current intake. This should bring the total intake to about 40 grams a day, or the amount a typical vegetarian eats.

However, it is not recommended that you try to double your intake of fiber overnight. Excess fiber can cause gas, a bloated feeling and diarrhea, problems that can be avoided by adding fiber to the diet gradually. Adding fiber to the diet may also reduce the quantities of nutrients the digestive tract can absorb from food, so be sure your diet is adequate in all other respects before increasing your fiber intake.

Work on the mineral selenium has shown that it too may be a cancer fighter. Variations in the geographical distribution of selenium have been associated with differences in cancer rates. A number of animal studies strongly support these human findings. Despite the encouraging results, the National Academy of Sciences does not feel the data are sufficient to prove that selenium will reduce your cancer risk. However, if you do choose to take a selenium supplement, the commonly available 50-microgram tablet of selenium would be a reasonable addition to your diet, since the daily human requirement is estimated to be between 50 and

200 micrograms. Daily intake of more than 500 micrograms, however, is potentially hazardous.

Two potential cancer preventers found only in certain processed foods are the preservatives BHT and BHA. On the basis of animal studies, it appears that the two micrograms of these food additives that the average American consumes each day may already be protecting Americans against cancer. In fact, some scientists have suggested that the low incidence of stomach cancer in the United States may be at least partly due to the widespread consumption of BHT and BHA in processed foods over the past several decades. However, it must be emphasized that the only direct evidence that these chemicals prevent cancer has been derived from work with laboratory animals. Until more controlled work with humans is attempted, we can only make a well-educated guess about their value to human beings.

While as a group Americans could probably benefit from eating more vitamin C, more vitamin A, more fiber and, perhaps, more selenium, it is equally true that we eat too much fat. We need only about a tablespoon of fat a day to stay healthy; many of us eat several times that much. There is a substantial amount of evidence that has linked diets high in fat with a higher susceptibility to cancers of the colon and breast. Animal studies tell us that fats can also increase the carcinogenic potential of many substances, including diethylstilbestrol (DES). Unsaturated fats are more likely than saturated fats to promote cancer, at least in animal studies. But saturated fats are believed to increase one's risk of heart disease. It has been suggested that the type of fat you eat should be based on your hereditary predisposition to either cancer or heart disease. However, this conclusion has not been adequately tested with controlled human trials.

The prescriptions we've noted above—eating vitamin C with nitrite-containing foods, eating lots of vegetables with carotene, eating more fiber and eating less fat all may work individually to reduce your susceptibility to environmental hazards. But can combining these individual behaviors into a dietary regime offer the body even greater protection? That question is nearly impossible to answer, since little research specifically evaluating the interaction of various parts of diet has been attempted. However, it is known that certain population groups that eat low- or no-meat, high-vegetable and high-fiber diets do seem to enjoy a lower risk of cancer than other Americans. For example, the Seventh-Day Adventists, many of whom follow a vegetarian lifestyle, have a markedly lower incidence of colon and breast cancers—two big killers. Vegetarians have been found to have fewer mutagens in their feces than most people, which may be related to their lower incidence of digestive tract cancer.

You do not, of course, have to become a vegetarian or change your religion to enjoy some of the benefits of these lifestyles. By eating more vegetables, fruits, whole-grain products and other foods rich in vitamin A, vitamin C and fiber, you should be able to reduce your chances of getting cancer. If you want to reduce your odds still further, consume less red meat and substitute instead more chicken and fish. When you do eat meat, cook it at lower temperatures, for example by broiling it or baking it in a moderate oven. A substantial quantity of mutagens is produced when meat is cooked until very well done at high temperatures. If you eat any cured meats, such as bacon or ham, drink orange juice or eat an orange beforehand.

These suggestions are meant for people of all ages, but they are especially relevant for parents of young children. Eating habits are formed early. The common dislike of vegetables and fruits, for example, usually begins in childhood, so try to set a good example for your children by eating good foods yourself. In particular, be sure your children get enough minerals. Calcium, phosphorus, copper, iron and magnesium deficiencies, as we mentioned earlier, can increase the absorption and toxicity of lead. Emphasize the use of fresh and frozen vegetables over those sold in cans with lead seals. Serve foods high in vitamin C if nitrites are included in the meal and put cooked vegetables in the refrigerator right after meals to keep the nitrates naturally found in vegetables from being converted to nitrites by bacteria, which can happen at room temperature.

Throughout this book, we have referred to the RDAs, or Recommended Dietary Allowances, of nutrients. These are standards set by the National Research Council and are designed to promote the growth, maintenance and reproductive functions of the human organism. They do not, however, consider the nature of nutrient-pollutant interactions or the extent to which dietary factors affect the occurrence of environmentally induced disease. It is our judgment that the concept of the RDA is sufficiently broad to incorporate this newly discovered function of nutrients. Future research by the National Research Council and the Food and Drug Administration should probably focus on reevaluating the RDAs in light of this knowledge.

One way to expedite this research might be to establish a federal research center devoted to studying nutrient-pollutant interactions. This center should be funded by the FDA, the Environmental Protection Agency and the National Institute for Occupational Safety and Health, since all of these agencies deal with various aspects of nutrition and hazards in the environment. Unfortunately, since no one agency now is responsible for looking both at nutrition and at environmental hazards—and at how those two interact—nutrient-pollutant interactions are falling in the cracks, as far as the government is concerned.

If diet can play a major role in preventing environmental disease, we need to know that as soon as possible. Earlier in this book, we noted that 25 percent of all Americans will get cancer in their lifetime and 70 percent of those people will die from cancer. That is a terrible toll we pay for our modern way of life. Perhaps, through proper nutrition, future generations will face far better odds.

By following the suggestions in this book, we believe you can live a healthier life. But health, that elusive state of physical well-being we all strive for, is the product of many variables, of which nutrition is only one. Heredity, age, occupation and even geographical location all help determine whether we will lead happy, healthy lives or succumb to illness. In this book we have shown that the environment is the source of many of the diseases that plague our society and that nutrition can prove to be a valuable tool in the fight against those diseases. We have not meant to suggest that by eating properly you will never get sick, only that nutrition is one of the ways you can better your odds of living to a healthy, ripe old age. And, living as we do in a veritable sea of hazardous agents, we need all the help we can get.

References |

General

Calabrese, Edward J. 1978. *Pollutants and High-Risk Groups: The Biological Basis of Increased Human Susceptibility to Environmental and Occupational Pollutants.* N.Y.: John Wiley and Sons.

Calabrese, Edward J. 1980, 1981. *Nutrition and Environmental Health: The Influence of Nutritional Status on Pollutant Toxicity and Carcinogenicity,* Vols. 1 and 2. N.Y.: John Wiley and Sons.

Fraumeni, J. F. 1975. *Persons at High Risk of Cancer: An Approach to Cancer Etiology and Control.* N.Y.: Academic Press.

Fritsch, Albert Q., ed. 1978. *The Household Pollutants Guide.* Garden City, N.Y.: Anchor Books.

Key, M. M., *et al.,* eds. 1977. *Occupational Diseases: A Guide to Their Recognition.* Washington, D.C.: U.S. Department of Health, Education and Welfare.

National Academy of Sciences. 1982. *Diet, Nutrition and Cancer.* Washington, D.C.: National Academy of Sciences Press.

Newell, G. R., and Ellison, N. M. 1981. *Nutrition and Cancer: Etiology and Treatment.* N.Y.: Raven Press.

Chapter 2

Culliton, Barbara J. 1977. "Saccharin: A Chemical in Search of an Industry." *Science* 196: 1179–1183.

Hecht, Annabel. 1978. "Aerosol Antiperspirants: Under a Cloud." *FDA Consumer* (November), pp. 10–11.

Hoffman, Eva, and Slade, Margot. 1982. "More on Coffee and Pregnancy." *New York Times* (January 24).

Kolata, Gina B. 1981. "Fetal Alcohol Advisory Debated." *Science* 214: 642–645.

McCamm, Michael. 1979. *Artist Beware.* N.Y.: Watson-Guptill Publications.

"NAS Saccharin Study Released." 1978/1979. *FDA Consumer* (December 1978/January 1979).

Putzrath, R. M., Langley, D., and Eisenstadt, E. 1981. "Analysis of Mutagenic Activity in Cigarette Smokers' Urine by High Performance Liquid Chromatography." *Mutation Research* 85: 97–108.

Rosenkranz, H. S. 1982. "Diesel Emissions and Health" (letter to the editor). *Science* 216: 360–362.

Shelby, M. D., and Taijiro, M. 1981. "Mutagens and Carcinogens in the Diet and Digestive Tract." *Mutation Research* 85: 177–183.

Stich, H. F., *et al.* 1981. "Clastogenic Activity of Caramel and Caramelized Sugars." *Mutation Research* 91: 129–136.

"Study Links Talc Use to Ovarian Cancer." 1982. *Boston Globe*, Associated Press (August 6), p. 3.

Sulik, K. K., Johnston, M. C., and Webb, M. A. 1981. "Fetal Alcohol Syndrome: Embryogenesis in a Mouse Model." *Science* 214: 936–938.

"TGA Level: The Chips Aren't Down." 1980. *Science News* (June 7).

Tokiwa, H., Nakagawa, R., and Ohnishi, Y. 1981. "Mutagenic Assay of Aromatic Nitro Compounds with *Salmonella typhimurium.*" *Mutation Research* 91: 321–325.

Chapter 3

Brody, Jane. 1981. *Jane Brody's Nutrition Book.* N.Y.: W. W. Norton.

DiPalma, J. R., and Ritchie, D. M. 1977. "Vitamin Toxicity." *Annual Review of Pharmacology and Toxicology* 17: 133–148.

Lafond, M. G., and Calabrese, E. J. 1979. "Is the Selenium Drinking Water Standard Justified?" *Medical Hypothesis* 5(8): 877–899.

Mertz, W. 1981. "The Essential Trace Elements." *Science* 213: 1332–1338.

"A Primer on Dietary Minerals." 1974. *FDA Consumer* (September).

"Some Facts and Myths of Vitamins." 1979. *FDA Consumer* (September).

Chapter 4

Ames, Bruce N. 1978. *Environmental Chemicals Causing Cancer and Genetic Birth Defects: Developing a Strategy to Minimize Human Exposure.* California Policy Seminar, Monograph No. 2. Berkeley: Institute of Governmental Studies, University of California.

Cassarett, Louis J., and Doull, John. 1975. *Toxicology: The Basic Science of Poisons.* N.Y.: Macmillan.

Hoffmann, G. R. 1982. "Mutagenicity Testing in Environmental Toxicology." *Environmental Science and Technology* 16: 560A–574A.

MacMahon, Brian, Pugh, Thomas, and Ipsen, Johanes. 1960. *Epidemiologic Methods*. Boston: Little, Brown.

Maugh, Thomas H., and Mark, Jean L. 1975. *Seeds of Destruction: The Science Report on Cancer Research*. N.Y.: Plenum Press.

Ruddon, Raymond W. 1981. *Cancer Biology*. N.Y.: Oxford University Press.

Weisburger, J. H., and Williams, G. M. 1981. "Carcinogen Testing: Problems and New Approaches." *Science* 214: 401–407.

Chapter 5

Blackstone, S., Hurley, R. J., and Hughs, R. E. 1974. "Some Inter-relationships Between Vitamin C (L-Ascorbic Acid) and Mercury in the Guinea Pig." *Food Cosmetics and Toxicology* 12: 511–516.

Cecil, H. C., *et al.* 1973. "Polychlorinated Biphenyl-Induced Decrease in Liver Vitamin A in Japanese Quail and Rats." *Bulletin of Environmental Contamination and Toxicology* 9(3): 179.

"DES in Feed: Promoting Growth—And Problems." 1979. *FDA Consumer* (May).

Dunning, W. F., Curtis, M. R., and Maun, M. E. 1949. "The Effect of Dietary Fat and Carbohydrate on Diethylstilbestrol-Induced Mammary Cancer in Rats." *Cancer Research* 9: 354–361.

Foy, H., *et al.* 1966. "Hepatic Injuries in Riboflavin and Pyridoxine Deficient Baboons—Possible Relations to Aflatoxin-Induced Hepatic Cirrhosis and Carcinoma in Africans." *Nature* 212: 150–153.

Mirvish, S. S. 1972. "Kinetics of N-nitrosation Reactions in Relation to Tumorigenesis Experiments with Nitrites Plus Amines or Ureas." In *N-nitroso Compounds: Analysis and Formation*. P. Boguveski, R. Preussmann, and E. A. Walker, eds., pp. 104–108. Lyon, France: International Agency for Research in Cancer.

Mirvish, S. S. 1975. "Blocking the Formation of N-nitroso Compounds with Ascorbic Acid *in Vitro* and *in Vivo*." *Annals of the New York Academy of Science* 258: 175–180.

Newberne, P. M., Rogers, A. E., and Wogan, G. W. 1968. "Hepato-renal Lesions in Rats Fed a Low Lipotrope Diet and Exposed to Aflatoxin." *Journal of Nutrition* 94: 331–334.

Newberne, P. M., and Young, V. R. 1966. "Effect of Diets Marginal in Methionine and Choline With and Without Vitamin B_{12} on Rat Liver and Kidney." *Journal of Nutrition* 89: 69.

Noller, K. L., and Fish, C. R. 1974. "Diethylstilbestrol Usage: Its Interesting Past, Important Present and Questionable Future." *Medical Clinics of North America* 58: 793–810.

Parizek, J., and Ostadalova, I. 1967. "The Protective Effect of Small

Amount of Selenite in Sublimate Intoxication." *Experientia* 23: 140–143.

Rodricks, Joseph V., Hesseltine, Clifford W., and Mehlman, Myron A., eds. 1977. *Myotoxins in Human and Animal Health.* Park Forest South, Ill.: Pathotox Publishers.

"Smoke with PCBs from Transformers Shuts Building." 1981. *Electrical World* (October), p. 30.

Tannenbaum, S. R., *et al.* 1978. "Nitrite and Nitrate Are Formed by Endogenous Synthesis in the Human Intestine." *Science* 200: 1487–1489.

Varghese, A. J., *et al.* 1978. "Non-volatile *N*-nitroso Compounds in Human Feces." In *Environmental Aspects of n-nitroso Compounds.* International Agency for Research on Cancer. IARC Scientific Publications No. 19, pp. 257–264.

Vauthey, M. 1951. "Protective Effect of Vitamin C Against Poisons. *Praxis* 40: 284–286.

Wagstaff, D. J., and Street, J. C. 1971. "Ascorbic Acid Deficiency and Induction of Hepatic Microsomal Hydroxylative Enzymes by Organochlorine Pesticides." *Toxicology and Applied Pharmacology* 19: 10–19.

Wattenberg, L. W. 1972. "Inhibition of Carcinogenic and Toxic Effects of Polycyclic Hydrocarbons by Phenolic Antioxidants and Ethoxyquin." *Journal of the National Cancer Institute* 48: 1425–1430.

Wattenberg, L. W. 1975. "Effect of Dietary Constituents on the Metabolism of Chemical Carcinogens." *Cancer Research* 35: 3326–3331.

Wattenberg, L. W. 1976. "Inhibition of Chemical Carcinogens by Antioxidants and Some Additional Compounds." In *Fundamentals of Cancer Prevention,* S. Takayama and T. Sugimura, eds. University Park, Baltimore: Proceedings of the 6th International Symposium of the Princess Takamatsu Cancer Research Fund.

Wolff, A. H., and Ochme, F. W. 1974. "Carcinogenic Chemicals in Food as Environmental Health Issues." *Journal of the American Veterinary Medicine Association* 164: 623–628.

Chapter 6

Bonner, Raymond. 1981. "Toxic Dumping in Niagara River Is Reported." *New York Times* (October 11), p. 48.

Bushnell, P. J., and DeLuca, H. F. 1981. "Lactose Facilitates the Intestinal Absorption of Lead in Weanling Rats." *Science* 211: 61–63.

Calabrese, Edward J., *et al.,* eds. 1980. *Drinking Water and Cardiovascular Disease.* Park Forest South, Ill.: Pathotox Publishers.

"Cancer Rate Spurs Anxiety in Industrial Bay Area." 1982. *New York Times* (March 28).

"Children, Gardens . . . and Lead." 1981. *The Mother Earth News* (July/August), pp. 38–41.

Cohen, B. L. 1980. "Health Effects of Radon from Insulation of Buildings." *Health Physics* 39(6): 937–941.

Flanagan, P. R., *et al.* 1978. "Increased Dietary Cadmium Absorption in Mice and Human Subjects with Iron Deficiency." *Gastroenterology* 74: 841–846.

Fletcher, B. L., and Tappel, A. L. 1973. "Protective Effects of Dietary α-tocopherol in Rats Exposed to Toxic Levels of Ozone and Nitrogen Dioxide." *Environmental Resources* 6: 165–175.

Goyer, R. A., and Cherian, M. G. 1979. "Ascorbic Acid and EDTA Treatment of Lead Toxicity in Rats." *Life Sciences* 24: 433–438.

Hill, C. H., *et al.* 1963. "*In Vivo* Interactions of Cadmium with Copper, Zinc and Iron." *Journal of Nutrition* 80: 227–235.

"How Insulation Traps the Bad and the Good." 1979. *Business Week* (December 24).

Hueber, Albert L. 1978. "Childhood's Hidden Epidemic." *The Nation* (March 4).

Karpatkin, Rhoda A. 1981. "Memo to Members." *Consumer Reports* (September), p. 494.

Keough, Carol. 1981. "Lead on Tap." *Organic Gardening* (May), pp. 86–92.

Knox, Richard A. 1982. "Child Lead Poisoning: An Invisible Menace." A two-part series, *Boston Globe* (February 7 and 8).

Leaderer, B. P. 1982. "Air Pollutant Emissions from Kerosene Space Heaters." *Science* 218: 1113–1115.

"Lead Poisoning from Lead Paint: The End of the Road?" 1977. *Consumer Reports* (March).

Leverett, D. H. 1982. "Fluorides and the Changing Prevalence of Dental Caries." *Science* 217: 26–30.

Mahaffey, K. 1974. "Nutritional Factors Affecting Lead Toxicity." *Environmental Health Perspectives* 7: 107–112.

Mahaffey, K., and Goyer, R. A. 1970. "Experimental Enhancement of Lead Toxicity by Low Dietary Calcium." *Journal of Laboratory and Clinical Methods* 76: 933–942.

Marshall, E. 1982. "A Turnabout on EPA Lead Rules." *Science* (August 20), 217: 711.

Menzel, D. B., *et al.* 1975. "Prevention of Ozonide-Induced Heinze Bodies in Human Erythrocytes by Vitamin E." *Archives of Environmental Health* 30: 234–236.

Nash, Timothy. 1981. "Truth Decay." *New Republic* (May 2), pp. 12–15.

National Academy of Sciences. 1977. *Drinking Water and Health*. Washington, D.C.: National Academy of Sciences Printing and Publishing Office.

Needleman, H. L., *et al.* 1979. "Deficits in Psychologic and Classroom Performance of Children with Elevated Dentine Lead Levels." *New England Journal of Medicine* 300(13): 689–695.

Piver, W. T. 1977. "Environmental Transport and Transformation of Automotive-Emitted Lead." *Environmental Health Perspectives* 19: 247–259.

"The Pollution Hazards (of Kerosene Heaters)." 1982. *Consumer Reports* (October), pp. 504–507.

Sebastien, P., Bignon, J., and Martin, M. 1982. "Indoor Airborne Asbestos Pollution: From Ceiling and the Floor." *Science* 216: 1410–1413.

Snowdon, C. T., and Sanderson, B. A. 1974. "Lead Pica Produced in Rats." *Science* 183: 92–94.

Spivy-Fox, M. R., *et al.* 1971. "Effect of Ascorbic Acid on Cadmium Toxicity in the Young Coturnix." *Journal of Nutrition* 101: 1295–1306.

Whitaker, Ralph. 1982. "Air Quality in the Home." *EPRI Journal* (March), pp. 7–14.

"Wood: 42 Million Cords Go Up in Smoke." 1982. *Energy Daily* (September 1), p. 4.

Yao, J. S., Calabrese, E. J., and DiNardi, S. R. 1978. "Does Ambient Ozone Pose a Serious Public Health Concern as a Widespread Environmental Mutagen?" *Medical Hypothesis* 4: 165–172.

Chapter 7

Aleksandrowicz, J., Starek, A., and Moszczynski, P. 1977. "The Effect of Selenium on Peripheral Blood Picture in Rats Chronically Exposed to Benzene." *Work Medicine* 28(6): 453–459.

Forssman, S., and Frykholm, K. O. 1947. "Benzene Poisoning. II. Examination of Workers Exposed to Benzene with Reference to the Presence of Estersulfate, Muconic Acid, Urochrome A and Polyphenols in the Urine Together with Vitamin C Deficiency. Prophylactic Measures." *Acta. Med Scand.* 128: 256.

Health, C. W., Jr., Falk, H., and Creech, J. L., Jr. 1975. "Characteristics of Cases of Angiosarcoma of the Liver among Vinyl Chloride Workers in the U.S." *Annals of the New York Academy of Science* 246: 231–236.

Heppel, L. A., Highman, B., and Porterfield, V. T. 1946. "Toxicology of 1,2-dichloropropane (Propylene Dichloride). II. Influence of Dietary Factors on the Toxicity of Dichloropropane." *J. Pharm. and Exp. Ther.* 87: 11–17.

Hoye, E. L. 1953. "The Toxicity of Tri-o-cresyl Phosphate for Rats as Related to Dietary Casein Levels, Vitamin E and Vitamin A." *Journal of Nutrition* 50: 609–622.

Kaw, J. L., Zaidi, S. H., and Path, F. C. 1969. "Effect of Ascorbic Acid on Pulmonary Silicosis of Guinea Pigs." *Archives of Environmental Health* 19: 74–82.

Lurie, J. B. 1965. "Benzene Intoxication and Vitamin C." *Occupational Med. Trans.* 16: 78–79.

Margolis, A. M., and Bakanova, G. D. 1966. "The Influence of Vitamin C Addition to a Routine Diet on the Human Organism Exposed to Occupational Hazards (in Presence of Intensive Sound Stimuli)." *Voprosy Pitaniia* 25: 34–38.

Mitchell, W. G., and Floyd, E. P. 1954. "Ascorbic Acid and Ethylene Diamine Tetraacetate as Antidotes in Experimental Vanadium Poisoning." *Proceedings of the Society of Experimental Biology and Medicine.* 85: 206–208.

Samitz, M. H., and Katz, S. 1965. "Protection Against Inhalation of Chromic Acid Mist: Use of Filters Impregnated with Ascorbic Acid." *Archives of Environmental Health* 11: 770–772.

Samitz, M. H. 1970. "Ascorbic Acid in the Prevention and Treatment of Toxic Effects from Chromates." *Acta. Dermatovener* 50: 59–64.

Shaver, S. L., and Mason, K. E. 1951. "Impaired Tolerance to Silver in Vitamin E Deficient Rats." *Anat. Rec.* 109: 382.

Viscount Chetwynd. 1917. "In Discussion on the Origin, Symptoms, Pathology, Treatment and Prophylaxis of Toxic Jaundice Observed in Munitions Workers." *Proc. Roy. Soc. Med.* 10: 6.

Young, T. B., Kananek, M. S., and Tsiatis, A. A. 1981. "Epidemiological Study of Drinking Water Chlorination and Wisconsin Female Cancer Mortality." *Journal of the National Cancer Institute* 67(6): 1191–1198.

Chapter 8

Altman, L. K. 1982. "Aspirin's Use in Preventing Heart Attacks Reported." *New York Times* (November 16), p. C3.

"Aspirin Diet Is Found to Slow Cancer in Rats." 1982. *New York Times,* Associated Press (April 18).

"Aspirin May Slow Advance of Cataracts, Professor Says." 1982. *Boston Globe,* Associated Press (February 14).

Baker, C. E., Jr., pub. 1982. *Physicians' Desk Reference*. Oradell, N.J.: Medical Economics Company.

Boston Women's Health Book Collective. 1976. *Our Bodies, Ourselves*. N.Y.: Simon and Schuster.

Calabrese, E. J. 1979. "Conjoint Use of Laetrile and Megadoses of Ascorbic Acid in Cancer Treatment: Possible Side Effects." *Medical Hypothesis* 5: 995–997.

Calabrese, E. J. 1979a. "Possible Adverse Side Effects from Treatment with Laetrile." *Medical Hypothesis* 5: 1045–1049.

Editors of Consumer Reports Books. 1980. *The Medicine Show*. New York: Pantheon Books.

Gal, I., Parkinson, C., and Craft, I. 1971. "Effects of Oral Contraceptives on Human Plasma Vitamin A Levels." *British Medical Journal* 2: 436–438.

Loh, H. S., Watters, K. J., and Wilson, C. W. M. 1974. "The Effects of Aspirin on the Metabolic Availability of Ascorbic Acid on Human Beings." *Journal of Clinical Pharmacology* 13: 480–486.

"The Pill May Limit a Cancer." 1982. *Boston Globe*, Associated Press (June 18).

Roe, Daphne. 1976. *Drug Induced Nutritional Deficiencies*. Westport, Conn.: The AVI Publishing Company.

Sahud, M. A., and Cohen, R. J. 1971. "Effect of Aspirin Ingestion on Ascorbic Acid Levels in Rheumatoid Arthritis." *Lancet* 1: 937–938.

Slade, Margot, and Hoffman, Eva. 1982. "Laetrile Verdict: It's the Pits." *New York Times* (January 31).

Taylor, Flora. 1980–1981. "Aspirin: America's Favorite Drug." *FDA Consumer* (December 1980/January 1981).

Wilson, C. W. M. 1975. "Clinical Pharmacological Aspects of Ascorbic Acid." In Second Conference on Vitamin C, C. G. King and J. J. Burns, eds., *Annals of the New York Academy of Science* 258: 355–376.

Chapter 9

Armstrong, B. K., *et al.* 1981. "Diet and Reproductive Hormones: A Study of Vegetarian and Non-vegetarian Postmenopausal Women." *Journal of the National Cancer Institute* 67(4): 761–767.

Brass, H. J., Weisner, M. J., and Kingsley, B. A. 1981. "Community Water Supply Survey: Sampling and Analysis for Purgeable Organics and Total Organic Carbon." Presented at the American Water Works Association Annual Meeting, Water Quality Division, June 6.

Burkitt, D. P., Walker, A. R., and Painter, N. S. 1972. "Effect of Dietary Fiber on Stools and Transit Times, and Its Role in the Causation of Disease." *Lancet* 2: 1408–1412.

Chowdhury, P., *et al*. 1982. "Cadmium-Induced Pulmonary Injury in Mouse: A Relationship with Serum Antitrypsin Activity." *Bulletin of Environmental Contamination and Toxicology* 28: 446–451.

Chu, E. W., and Malmgren, R. A. 1965. "An Inhibitory Effect of Vitamin A in the Induction of Tumors of Forestomach and Cervix in the Syrian Hamster by Carcinogenic Polycyclic Hydrocarbons." *Cancer Research* 25: 884–895.

Davison, K. L., Sell, J. L., and Rose, R. J. 1970. "Dieldrin Poisoning of Chickens During Severe Dietary Restriction." *Bulletin of Environmental Contamination and Toxicology* 5: 493–501.

Ellis, K. J., *et al*. 1979. "Cadmium: *In Vivo* Measurement in Smokers and Non-smokers." *Science* 205: 323–325.

Fujimaki, Y. 1926. "Formation of Gastric Carcinoma in Albino Rats Fed on Deficient Diets." *Cancer Research* 10:469.

Gunby, P. 1978. "Retinoid Chemoprevention Trial Begins Against Bladder Cancer." *Journal of the American Medical Association* 240(7): 609.

Hankin, J. H., and Rawlings, V. 1978. "Diet and Breast Cancer: A Review." *American Journal of Clinical Nutrition* 31: 2005–2016.

Mushett, C. W., *et al*. 1952. "Antidotal Efficacy of Vitamin B_{12} (Hydroxocobalamin) in Experimental Cyanide Poisoning." *Proceedings of the Society of Experimental Biology and Medicine* 81: 254–257.

Pearce, M. L., and Dayton, S. 1971. "Incidence of Cancer in Men on a Diet High in Polyunsaturated Fat." *Lancet* 1: 464–467.

Phillips, R. L. 1975. "Role of Life-Style and Dietary Habits in Risk of Cancer Among Seventh-Day Adventists." *Cancer Research* 35: 3513–3522.

Shekelle, R. B., *et al*. 1981. "Dietary Vitamin A and Risk of Cancer in the Western Electric Study." *Lancet* 2 (8257): 1185–1190.

Smith, A. D. M., Duckett, S., and Waters, A. H. 1963. "Neuropathological Changes in Chronic Cyanide Intoxication." *Nature* 200: 179–181.

Sporn, M. B., *et al*. 1977. "13-*cis*-retinoic Acid: Inhibition of Bladder Carcinogenesis in the Rat." *Science* 195: 487–489.

Stantchev, von St., *et al*. 1979. "Administration of Granular Pectin to Workers Exposed to Lead." *Zeit. Ges. Hygiene Grenzgebiet* 25: 585–587.

United States Environmental Protection Agency. 1982. "National Revised Primary Drinking Water Regulations, Volatile Synthetic Organic Chemicals in Drinking Water; Advanced Notice of Proposed Rulemaking." *Federal Register* 47(3): 9350–9358.

Wechsler, I. S. 1933. "Etiology of Polyneuritis." *Arch. Neurol. Psychiat.* 29: 813.

Wilson, R., and DeEds, E. F. 1950. "Importance of Diet in Studies of Chronic Toxicity." *Archives of Industrial Hygiene and Occupational Medicine* 1: 73–80.

Wynder, E. L., *et al.* 1969. "Environmental Factors of Cancer of the Colon and Rectum: II Japanese Epidemiological Data. *Cancer* 23(5): 1210–1220.

Index